NEW

BOOK

on

Healing

by
Rev. Hanna Kroeger

"My people are dying from lack of knowledge."

This phrase from the Bible means that in order for us to take advantage of the healing power that lies within each one of us, we have to cooperate with nature and allow God's miracle foods and herbs to do their work. Instinctively we know we must return to nature to heal ourselves. So let this book become a guidepost on your healing journey.

The help contained within these pages is time proven. The simple message allows each one of us to take an active role in healing ourselves and our families. Herewith I give you "new" ways to continue helping each other.

This book will give guidance. However, if you have a medical problem, this knowledge is no substitute for medical help.

Book available at: Hanna's Herb Shop
5684 Valmont Road
Boulder, Colorado 80301
(800) 206-6722
(303) 443-0755   Fax (303) 938-9021

Please call to confirm before mailing.
Visa, MasterCard, and money orders only please.

ISBN 1-883713-17-X
© 1996 by Hanna Kroeger Publications

New Book on Healing
by Hanna Kroeger

~ Acne ~

*see also Dermatitis, Eczema, Skin

For facial acne, try Homeopathic *Bellis perennris* (daisy).

A home remedy for acne is buttermilk and honey: Boil the buttermilk. When thickened, add the honey so it becomes a thick cream. Apply to the face or wherever there is an acne problem.

~ Alcoholism ~

To combat alcoholism, the following recipes may help:

Chromium and vanadium mixed together, one teaspoon two times daily, will reduce the desire for alcohol.

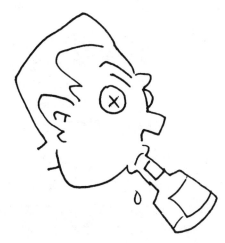

Sometimes there are parasites in the pancreas in alcoholic cases. Therefore, Homeopathic "Pancreatic Flukes" might help.

Liver Rebuilder:

I found the following recipe in an old book used in 1802 by Dr. Selig of Austria. It sounded so good that I tried it and found that it is truly excellent.

Boil: 1 teaspoon dandelion root
      1 teaspoon angelica or arnica
      1 teaspoon wormwood
      1 teaspoon gentian

Simmer in two cups water & strain. Add 2 quarts apple juice and 4 ounces freshly squeezed lemon juice, and drink this in small portions during the day. Do this for 2–3 days and repeat if needed once a month. Take only stewed fruit and apple juice on these days.

Take 1 tablespoon Epsom salts in the morning and one at night.

The herb ginkgo biloba is a tremendous help for alcohol cravings.

Alcoholics also suffer from severe vitamin C, vitamin B, and zinc deficiencies.

– Allergies –

When the body detects a foreign substance, it will react in what is called "allergies," or sometimes it is called "hayfever." The common symptoms are runny noses, itching eyes, a burning sensation in the lungs, etc. There are several ways to relieve allergy symptoms, including:

Wild plum bark syrup.

Orange rind or peelings, mixed in a tea, is helpful for allergy symptoms.

Honey—what we call "the ambrosia of the gods." Each area within a country has its own distinctive type of honey. It is said that to relieve allergy symptoms you should use honey from your own neighborhood. It can act as an antihistamine.

Allergies and hayfever are symptoms of toxins and poisons in the bloodstream, of the lymphatic system and the tissues. Every ½ hour drink 4 ounces of pure water. Do this for 2 days. Then make yourself a vegetable broth and drink on the full hour 6 ounces of broth and on the ½ hour 4 ounces of water.

Orange rind or peelings is such a good allergy reliever. The stuffed-up nose and clogged-up air passages open up and healthful sleep can be expected.

All allergies have two factors in common: chemical poison and parasites. See a physician to find *your parasites.*

– Anemia –

The following recipes will help the anemic sufferers rebuild their systems:

Red beets are good for anemia, leukemia, and septic blood.

Egg yolk mixed in concord grape juice is an excellent blood builder.

Blackstrap molasses is a mineral and iron supplier.

Lentils contain protein supplies and iron of the best quality.

Grapes are good for anemia and to build the aura.

Spinach is tremendously helpful in anemic cases.

Red beets can contribute substantially to an anemic. Raw juice: take only 2 tablespoons 4 times daily. Raw beet and apple salad with onions is superb. Boiled beet as soup (Borscht) is Russia's favorite. Beet salad from cooked beets or pickled beets is also used.

Eggplant increases red blood cells, improving anemia. It is also known as a good tonic. If eggplant is sliced and placed in lightly salted water for about 20 minutes, the bitter taste will be alleviated.

~ Angina ~

*see also Arteries, Circulation
Problems, Heart Disease

What symptoms does your body give you when plaque is building up in the arteries?

1) Watch for an overly tired feeling after a heavy meal.
2) Observe forgetfulness with tasks which you normally perform with acuity.
3) Notice if your mind will not grasp new ideas or follow new dimensions.
4) Persistent feeling of weakness, coldness, tingling, or burning in your toes or feet.
5) Be aware of dull headaches.
6) Persistent sleeplessness is another danger signal.
7) Tightness in chest.
8) Pain in shoulders, if not accident related.
9) Breathlessness when walking or lifting.
10) Notice if walking gives you pain in the calves of the legs, and if when you rest you feel better and pain disappears.
11) Notice: You had a good night's sleep. You get up and stretch or exercise. In the middle of the sternum is a sharp pain. It will go away and not return until next morning when the same pain returns at the same time in the middle of the sternum.
12) Notice if there are small ulcerations of your skin on ankles or feet.

The answer is *Aurum metallicum* and *Spigelia anthelmia* in Homeopathic form. Also Circu Flow.

– Anorexia Nervosa –

Anorexia nervosa is a refusal to eat, causing a severe weight loss. This condition usually begins during the teenage years. They have a distorted view of their bodies as being too fat, even after they have lost a large percentage of their body weight.

Although most anorexic cases are psychologically based, some studies suggest that there is a *zinc deficiency* causing the problem or making it worse. Some good sources of zinc in the diet are: lean meat, poultry, fish, shellfish, oatmeal, whole wheat bread, peas, lima beans, egg yolks, brewer's yeast, wheat germ, milk, and yogurt.

Cloves help to stimulate the appetite, making it easier for the anorexic to recover.

Rub your earlobes several times a day.

~ Anxiety ~

*see also Nervous Conditions

When a person has a great deal of anxiety, they need chromium and magnesium. Borage and thyme tea are also good for anxiety.

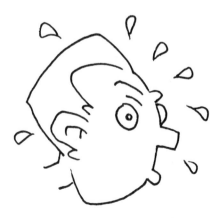

~ **Appetite** ~

*see also Sugar Craving

When there is a loss of appetite, eating apples helps to regain it.

Alfalfa in small amounts creates sound appetite and improves digestion.

Caraway, a very well known spice, and eggplant both help improve the appetite as well.

Feeding oatmeal to children is said to stimulate their appetite, which can be useful when a child is not flourishing. Oatmeal is also extremely healing internally and may be used by any invalid during any convalescence.

The homeopathic remedy that helps when there is a loss of appetite is *Taraxacum officinale* (dandelion).

When a person has too large of an appetite, they need enzymes with their meals.

~ **Arms** ~

When there are nodules in the arm, Homeopathic *Hippozaurium* helps.

When there is pain in the left upper arm, watch the heart. Sometimes the muscle in the arms hurt because arsenic poisoning has settled in the muscles.

~ Arteries ~

*see also Angina, Circulation
Problems, Heart Disease

Aloe vera aids in assimilation, circulation, and elimination. It has been reported to increase endurance and energy and to provide a speedy recovery from fatigue. To clean your arteries, take the herbal chelation formula along with aloe vera gel.

Aloe vera is not a drug. It does not react with medications. Some properties in aloe vera are as follows:

Active Ingredients:	Minerals:	Vitamins:
Amino acids	Calcium	A
Enzymes	Magnesium	E
Natal aloes	Sodium	K
Aloin	Potassium	B_1
Emodin	Strontium	B_2
Bitter resins	Boron	B_3
Barbaloin	Silicon	B_6
Chlorophyll	Copper	Folic Acid
Albumin	Manganese	Choline
Essential oils	Iron	
Gum arabic	Aluminum	
Silica	Lithium	
Phosphate of Zinc	Nickel	
	Zinc	

Other agents of aloe vera:
Pain killer, fungicidal, germicidal, virucidal, anti-inflammatory (similar to steroid effects), anti-pyretic (reduces fever and heat of sores), anes-

thetizes tissue, natural cleanser, penetrates tissue, dilates capillaries, breaks down and digests dead tissue, including pus (through proteolytic enzymes—degenerative stage of sickness), enhances normal cell proliferation—regenerative stage of healing, reduces bleeding time.

– Arthritis –

Epsom salts are useful to relieve pain in the hands and feet, especially after a sprain or with arthritis. Put about 1 tablespoon of Epsom salts in warm water and soak for about 20 minutes.

Flax seed contains a remarkable healing oil which can be used externally or internally. Flax oil is useful for arthritis.

Apple cider vinegar, honey, and water, together, have been used for thousands of years by many different cultures to "balance" the body. This combination has also been found to be extremely beneficial to people with arthritic pain when taken every morning. It has been known to restore supple movement in hands and dissolve knots. The recipe is 2 teaspoons apple cider vinegar, 2 teaspoons honey, and 8 ounces water. Take it 3 times daily with meals.

Swiss chard is wonderful for arthritis because it contains Wulzen factor.

Another great recipe for relieving arthritis is 1 tablespoon whey, 1 tablespoon lecithin in juice, 2 times daily.

Make a tea of the herb willow bark. Try to relax, as tension and stress aggravate pain. Praying or meditating might help as well. ⬎

~ **Asthma** ~

***see also Bronchial Trouble,
Bronchitis, Cough, Lung**

Cranberry juice should be drunk on a regular basis by people suffering from asthma. Use concentrated cranberry juice when an asthma attack is imminent: Put ½ teaspoon or less of the cranberry concentrate on the inside of the bottom lip. Use only a small amount so that the person will not choke. This might snap the person out of the attack immediately. You may buy the concentrated cranberry juice at your health food store, or you may prepare it yourself: One pound cranberries and one pint water boiled together until cranberries are done. Store in the refrigerator.

Another method to relieve a person from asthma is to soak two pieces of cloth in apple cider vinegar and wrap around each wrist, secured with plastic wrap.

Wild plum tree bark is wonderful for asthma. Make a syrup from it and take 1 tablespoon 4 times a day. You may also make a pillow from the bark to sleep with it.

For bronchial asthma, angelica root tea with honey will help.

Old asthmatic cases love anise tea, and it has been found to be useful for relieving asthma.

Cinnamon has been helpful for asthma, wheezing and coughing.

Grate black radish and add honey to it. Take one teaspoon of this mixture before going to bed to help with asthma.

For asthma, go on a ½-day fast. The time you do not eat, drink 2 quarts of water. Soak fresh pineapples in 2 quarts of water for two hours. Drink from this fluid for the other half of the day. Do this for 10–14 days.

One teaspoon of thyme powder mixed with honey taken every hour has helped some asthma cases.

Lemon juice, 2 tablespoons before each meal, will help alleviate asthma.

Sunflower seeds are nature's remedy for asthma: Take one quart of seeds, put in a half gallon of water and boil down to one quart of water. Strain, add one pint of honey, and then boil it down to a syrup. Give one teaspoon three times a day.

Asthma in children is best treated with Homeopathic Thuja and cranial work.

Cranial Work:

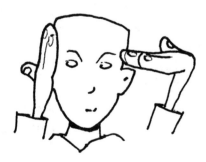

Lift bones on left side of head. Hold for 45 seconds. Do that 2 times daily. In a few days, asthma caused by anxiety will leave. Children often need only 1 treatment.

The homeopathic remedy for adults with asthma is *Eriodictyon glutinosum* (yerba santa).

When a person has asthma because of nervousness, have them take dandelion root and leaves tea.

For asthma without anxiety, take ginger.

Wild cherry bark is also good for asthma. ⤝

~ Attention Deficit Disorder ~

*see also Hyperactivity

Attention Deficit Disorder (ADD) affects 3.5 million American children (mostly males). Though often misdiagnosed, it stands as the most common behavioral disorder in American children. Medical experts agree that three characteristics show up in most cases:

1) distractibility
2) impulsive behavior
3) hyperactivity

Also, the disorder can be recognized in these modes of behavior:

• a short attention span (especially for low-interest activities)
• poor endings after enthusiastic beginnings
• low frustration tolerance and difficulty listening

- argumentative, and frequent job changes
- underachievement, in relation to ability
- frequent mood swings, and unpredictable
- avoids group activities, often labeled as a "loner"

What causes this condition?

A defect in the frontal lobes of the brain that is genetically passed explains some cases. Scientists also have considered outside factors such as: arsenic, dioxins, preservatives, environmental toxins, food dyes, and chemical additives. These have definitely been implicated as causal factors in ADD.

The underlying cause of ADD is extremely important to understand because it not only involves the chemical factors, but it has spiritual implications as well. Every child would have the behavior disorders that distinguish ADD if this were not true. When a child has some type of spiritual trauma at a young age (even when still in the womb), this breaks the protective shield around the nervous system, so that it is vulnerable to chemical poisons.

What can be used to counteract the environmental poisons? Often-prescribed stimulants such as ritalin, cylert, and dexedrine do not address these and cannot counteract accumulated poisons.

"New Light on ADD," though it has no curative properties, may assist the body in structure and function to defend itself against chemical and environmental invaders.

"Birthright Tea" heals the trauma. *Plumbum metallicum* is to clear the lead poisoning. "New Light" liquid helps eliminate the poisons.

Also, vitamin B_1 supplement will help in ADD sufferers.

~ Autism ~

A person who has autism is characterized as one who resists change, has repetitive acts and learning/speech disorders. Treatment for autism should include avoidance of sugar and food allergens. A good supplement should include calcium, magnesium, vitamin B_6, and chromium for the hypoglycemia.

Many autism sufferers have parasites in the pancreas. Take Homeopathic Pancreatic Flukes.

~ Aversion to Water ~

When a person has an aversion to water, homeopathic *Stramonium* (thorn apple) will help.

A lack of amino acids will cause a person to have an aversion to amino acids. Also lack of protein.

~ Bacterial Infections ~

Cabbage has been called the medicine of the poor and is extremely valuable for its healing qualities. Research indicates that cabbage contains ingredients which prevent cancer, making it an important addition to any diet. It is anti-inflammatory, antibacterial, and encourages new cell growth.

Onions have always been known to have anti-bacterial properties. Since onions easily absorb bacteria, they can be used in a sickroom to help disinfect it.

Goldenseal root (*Hydrastis canadensis*) is excellent in helping to combat bacterial infections.

Black pepper is thought to be one of nature's most perfect foods, as it both cures and prevents many diseases. It kills bacteria and can be used as a food preservative.

Garlic has been prized by healers for more than 5,000 years. Pyramid builders and Roman soldiers on long marches were given a daily ration of garlic. Garlic is so strong an antibiotic that the English purchased tons of it during World War I just for use on wounds. Journals of that period state that when garlic was used on wounds there were no cases of sepsis. It is a world-renowned cure-all and home remedy in practically every culture. Today, even orthodox medicine accepts its healing powers.

Cinnamon is a germicide, which will help with bacterial infections.

The fiber in whole-grain foods discourages the growth of harmful bacteria.

– Bad Breath –

When a person has bad breath, it sometimes can point to the disturbed function of the gall-bladder or the liver or both. It may also be a sign of major gum disease. Some diseases that can also cause bad breath include tuberculosis, syphilis, dehydration, and zinc deficiency.

Some home remedies that have worked to combat bad breath include sipping thyme tea or chewing on dill seeds to freshen the breath.

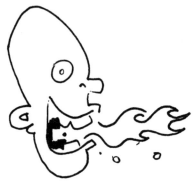

Caraway is very much like anise, and when they are both mixed together, they are twice as good. They help to sweeten the breath when chewed or as a tea.

The homeopathic remedy for bad breath is *Arsenicum Baptista.*

– Bed Wetting –

To help a child stop wetting the bed, you should try elevating the foot of the bed. Do not punish a child for wetting the bed, and try not to give a child potatoes for supper. Vitamin B_6 has also been helpful with this problem.

Cinnamon has been helpful to stop bed wetting, and it also helps children sleep at night.

The following teas have been helpful; however, serve them no later than 4 hours before they go to sleep: violet leaf tea, bistort tea, equisetum as a tea.

The homeopathic for bedwetting is *Calcerea phosporica*, and *Sepia* (cuttlefish).

Bedwetting can be the result of food sensitivities. Chromium and vanadium, calcium and magnesium, avoidance of sugar, simple sugars, and avoidance of allergenic foods have all been known to help stop bedwetting.

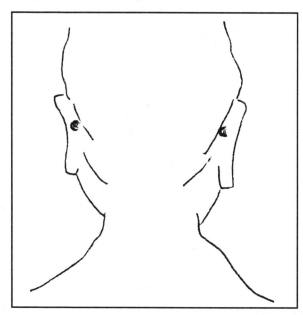

Behind the ears are two tiny holes. Massage these holes with a very light pressure. At the same time ask someone to rub the feet with a towel until they are warm.

~ Belching ~

To help stop belching, avoid carbonated beverages, eat slowly, avoid chewing gum, and avoid foods with high air content. Papaya tablets have an enzyme that will help stop you from belching.

Saw palmetto as a tea is a good remedy for belching, as well as massaging your earlobes.

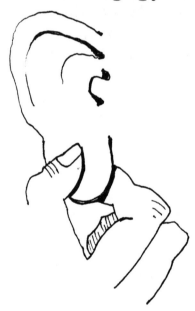

~ Bites ~

When you get bit by a mosquito, mix baking soda and cream of tartar with a little bit of water to make a paste, then apply it to your skin.

For other insect bites, make a tea of sage and then rub it on the affected area.

For a rattlesnake bite, wet some salt and wrap the bitten arm or leg in a salt pack, making sure the bite gets an extra dose of salt. Then RUSH to your physician!

If you get bitten by a dog or cat, assess the damage first in case you need to get medical attention. Then thoroughly wash the wound with soap and water to remove saliva and other contamination. Continue washing for 5 full minutes. Do not shy away from a tetanus shot. Take Homeopathic Thuja afterwards.

How to Remove Ticks:

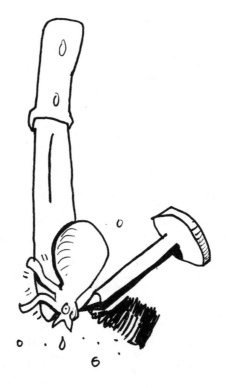

To remove ticks, take a large nail and heat the tip in a match flame. Slide the flat side of a knife blade under the tick's back so it is between the knife and the nail. When you see the tick's legs wiggle because it is getting too hot, turn the knife blade 90 degrees so the tick is standing on its head. Keeping it sandwiched, gently pull the tick up and away from its grip. If the legs do not wiggle, the nail is not warm enough. Try again. Once you've removed the tick, wash the bite area with soap and water, then apply iodine or another antiseptic to guard against infection. See your doctor!

Thyme tea has been used as a skin antiseptic for insect and snake bites.

Poisonous spider bites and insect bites need to be brought to the attention of your doctor, and the use of the homeopathic "Glondirine" will help as well.

To avoid getting bit by mosquitoes, use screen windows and doors. Electric bug zappers work well outdoors. Mosquitoes are not only irritating, they can carry a number of serious human diseases including meningitis, encephalitis, malaria, and yellow fever. Herbs like pennyroyal oil can be rubbed on the skin to repel insects. Taking vitamin B$_1$ at 500 mg daily may also help to repel mosquitoes.

~ **Bladder Infection** ~

To help heal a bladder infection, take a wool blanket and spread it on your bed. Place a cotton sheet over it, and sleep on it. It will also help with kidney problems.

Collinsonia root is good as a tea for a bladder infection, as well as drinking plenty of cranberry juice.

When you are having bladder trouble, take a pomegranate and juice it. Mix one half cup, with one half cup water, and sip it. It is even better as a fruit eaten two times a day.

When your bladder muscle is weak, pumpkin seed is terrific for strengthening the bladder muscle. Take one teaspoon three times daily or more if desired.

For bladder stones, drink parsley tea, one quart daily for three days, then just two cups a day for 2 weeks.

~ **Bleeding** ~

For bleeding, try either sesame oil, 2 teaspoons a day, or yarrow tea, 1 cup daily.

For intestinal bleeding, or bleeding under the skin, drink shepherd's purse tea, 1 cup twice a day.

Ice to the nipples will stop uterine bleeding. For excessive bleeding, contact your doctor at once.

Orange peeling tea is used to stop female hemorrhages.

See your doctor! ⤳

~ Blisters ~

When you have blisters in the palm of your hand, take homeopathic *Ranunculus bulbosus* (buttercup).

When you have blisters in your mouth, eat the spice sage, or make it into a tea.

Another method for ridding yourself of blisters in your mouth is to make a tea of arnica and violet and hold it in your mouth and drink it. ⤳

~ Bloated Condition ~

*see also Fluid Retention, Water-logged Tissues
Anise has been used for bloated conditions, especially in infants. Make a very diluted tea, and give a few drops in water as needed.

Fennel tea and sage tea have both had great success in bloated conditions.

Gentian is also a good tonic for bloated conditions: use ½ to 1 cup of gentian tea a day.

Be kind to your gallbladder. ⤳

~ Blood ~

*see also Blood Clotting
Your blood and platelets form an unwanted glue-like substance. If glue-like substances in the

blood are allowed to accumulate, the platelets release a dangerous waste called adenosine diphosphate, or ADP. Once ADP is released, other platelets glue together. They form clumps that obstruct the flow of blood through the vessel, and this may lead to blood clot in the heart (heart attack), the brain (stroke), the lung, or any other vital organs.

To decongest your blood the following recipes have worked for many:

Take some onions and cut them into pieces. Add to water and simmer to make onion water. White and red onions together have more anticlotting power. Drink ½ cup onion water 5 times daily and take 50 mg B$_6$ with each ½ cup of onion water. Bananas and tomatoes, rice and millet are allowed during this diet. Do this for 2 days in a row. Then pick up a good healthy diet, but continue with vitamin B$_6$.

Red clover leaf tea is excellent for the blood.

A mild blood cleanser is to take sanicle, 1 teaspoon to a cup of boiling water.

Another mild blood cleanser is to take 5 parts of red clover and 1 part of chaparral. Make a tea, and drink two cups daily.

A much stronger blood cleanser is to take 1 teaspoon of sassafras tea to a cup of boiling water.

One teaspoon sheep sorrel when added to a cup of boiling water is a strong blood cleanser as well.

When you take lemon juice, honey, and water and drink 6 ounces every 2 hours, it will help to decongest your blood.

Hyssop tea is a good blood purifier. Refer to the Bible: "Wash me with Hyssop and make me white as snow."

Rosemary is known as a blood thinner, and it also stimulates circulation.

To help blood circulate better, ground red pepper into your socks.

Egg yolk mixed in some concord grape juice is a terrific blood builder.

Carrots are good blood builders and contain vitamin A.

Watermelon seeds dilate the blood vessels, and also help to lower blood pressure.

Red beets are good for septic blood.

Bananas are loaded with potassium. We need potassium to keep the blood healthy.

Three homeopathic remedies for blood poisoning are *Baptisia tinctoria* (wild indigo), *Crataegus oxycantha* (hawthorn), and *Echinacea angustifolia* (cone flower).

~ Blood Clotting ~

*see also Blood

Parsley, carrots, broccoli, and citrus fruits all prevent blood clotting. The active food components in these are called "coumarins."

Rosemary has been known to be a blood thinner.

Blood Clots:

Have your friend comfortable on the bed or worktable. Flex his knees. Have his hands folded as in prayer, but his forefingers should form a pyramid. His thumbs close over it. There is nothing like a blanket pulled over you to give you more security. Now sit on his left side. Spread your arms out so that the right hand is over his head. The left hand is slipped under the cover. Hold it close to the tail bone. You cuddle your friend visibly and invisibly. Your hands do not touch the body at all but are one inch away from it.

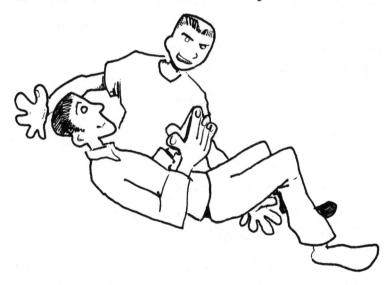

Now relax and tell your friend to do likewise. With all your heart concentrate on your work. Pray, and your energies will be poured into your friend's body. In case someone wants to help you, let him do so by touching your shoulders while standing behind you and also pouring energies through you into the patron's body.

Under your hands the miracle takes place. The blood becomes magnetically charged, and the blood clot disintegrates. Visibly the redness disappears, the breathing becomes easier, and the fever disappears. (The credit for this method goes to Rev. F.M. Houston.)

– Blood Pressure –

Potassium helps control high blood pressure.

For high blood pressure, mistletoe and angelica are excellent. Mix 2 teaspoons of each in one quart of water. Bring to a boiling point and drink 2–3 cups a day.

Garlic regulates blood pressure (so it can be used for both high and low blood pressure), and it is an anticoagulant, which means it may prevent strokes. It helps unclog arteries coated with plaque and is an aid in combating hypertension. The active food component in garlic is "gamma-glutamyl allylic cysteines."

The homeopathic remedy for high blood pressure is "Uranium Niticum," and the remedy for low blood pressure is "Cactus grandiflorus."

For high blood pressure, you need more potassium, preferably from fruits and vegetables such as peas and beans.

~ **Body Odor** ~

To combat body odor, drink tomato juice daily.

Parsley prevents body odor because of chlorophyll, a natural deodorant.

If you have very strong body odor, you need a liver remedy, which is homeopathic *Chelidonium majus* (celandine).

A good treatment for body odor is zinc, calcium/magnesium, plant derived colloidal minerals, lots of green leafy vegetables, and alfalfa.

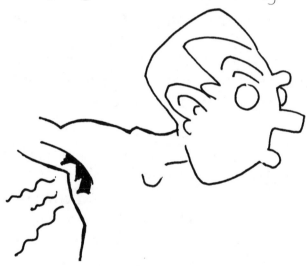

~ **Boils** ~

For boils, garden sage and corn meal as a poultice have worked very well.

Another remedy is to use a flaxseed poultice.

Boils are serious and often need the attention of your physician.

~ **Bone Problems** ~

Cabbage is very helpful in building up the bones.

Bananas are loaded with potassium, and we need potassium to keep bones healthy.

When you have bone, tendon, and muscle injuries, use comfrey root compresses, externally only.

When your bones are weak, take fenugreek seed in tablet or capsule form.

There is a virus named Coxsackie virus, a true enemy to the bones. It lodges first in the hip bones and then spreads to the entire bone system. Ask for homeopathic remedy "Coxsackie"; this is the only thing I know to do.

~ **Bowels** ~

To soothe the bowels, simmer flaxseed for about a half hour. Allow it to stand where it will remain hot for an hour or two longer. Put two tablespoonfuls in two cups of boiling water. Let it boil down to one cup. Add a little sugar to taste. The juice of half a lemon makes a tasty addition. Drink the whole cupful at bedtime, and swallow all the seeds. The mucilage is soothing to the bowels and, in combination with the seeds, often produces a good bowel movement. Excellent to take once a week, every four days, or more often as needed. Also, flax seed can be added to laxative formulas to prevent cramping of the bowels.

The tea of cinnamon bark, one half cup 4 times a day will heal all bleeding bowels. Another option is to chew on cinnamon bark until you can visit your physician.

Black pepper as a tea will help running bowels.

Barley is an excellent food for children suffering from inflammation of the bowels.

Alfalfa helps make the bowels move.

Always check for protozoa and worms.

~ Brain ~

*see also Forgetfulness, Memory

Dried apple peelings made into a tea are full of silicon and will help strengthen the brain.

Almonds are a good brain tonic. Almond oil, only 1 teaspoon daily, will improve your memory.

To strengthen your concentration, take more vitamin B_{12}, folic acid, and gotu kola.

Having rosemary tea every morning is thought to have restorative qualities and "comfort the brain."

To help children whose brain is slower than some, dill seeds and alfalfa seeds are thought to be beneficial.

Cloves in your tea will heighten your memory.

Oats have been known to be brain food.

Sage on a slice of very lightly buttered rye bread does wonders for the brain.

The meat of a coconut is brain food.

Eyebright in capsules or tablets helps strengthen the memory and the brain.

Cardamom is excellent for the brain.

To improve memory, take two mustard seeds.

Basil is food for the brain. When you feel victimized or criticized, eat some basil. If you wash your hands, arms, and face with basil tea, you can cope with an unfriendly world better.

When there is mental dullness, take hawthorn in tablets or as a tea.

Lemon balm has been used throughout history in preparations designed to promote youth. It is thought to strengthen the brain.

The homeopathic remedy for brain congestion is *Apis mellifica* (honey bee).

Mental Confusion:
Dulcamar or purple cone flower can be used for mental confusion.

~ Bronchial Trouble ~

***see also Asthma, Bronchitis, Cough,
Emphysema, Lung, Respiratory**
Yerba santa is an herb that may help when there is a bronchial infection.

When there is bronchial trouble, take thyme tea, 1 tablespoon every hour.

Mix dandelion leaves and fennel in equal parts and make a tea. Drink 3 to 4 cups a day to help with any type of bronchial trouble.

Cloves are also called Peruvian balm. Truly it is a balm if you have bronchial catarrh or other loud rattles in the chest. If you suffer from mucus in the chest or urine, cloves will benefit your condition. Take one cup of hot water and add a dash of cloves. If you want to add some honey, that is fine. This recipe will also help relieve nausea and vomiting.

Anise is a comforting antiseptic tea for colds and coughs. It can help bronchial problems.

~ Bronchitis ~

***see also Asthma, Bronchial Trouble,
  Cough, Lung, Respiratory**

Myrtle leaves contain Myrtal, an active antiseptic. It is used as a tea for bronchitis, coughing, cystitis, and helps when there is thick, yellow mucus.

Flax is helpful for bronchitis, and a tea made from the seeds is thought to help pulmonary infections. To make tea, brew the seeds in a pint of water, add the juice of two lemons, add three tablespoons of honey, and take a teaspoon every half hour until relieved.

If a person has bronchitis in their old age, white hellebore has been known to be helpful.

Myrrh can be used in chest rubs for congestion and bronchitis.

The following herbs have been known to be helpful for bronchitis: daffodil, lungwort, plantain, or H-12.

One thing that might easily be overlooked, intentionally or not, is that if you smoke, it is harder to overcome bronchitis.

For bronchitis, take the herb echinacea, either as a tea or in capsule form.

~ Bruises ~

If you bruise easily, you need more vitamin C, rutin, and bioflavonoids.

If you get a black eye, first pack it in ice so that the ice rests more to the forehead and to the cheekbones, so that the eye is not pressured. Also, champion boxers carry a small piece of iron with them in case of a black eye. They place the iron over the cheek and forehead and the bleeding or swelling stops.

For bruises, a handful of fresh crushed peach leaves applied as a poultice will help tremendously.

Salamon seal poultices or daisy tea poultices will also help relieve bruises.

Used as a poultice of hot milk and crushed seeds, fenugreek relieves bruises.

~ Burns ~

Aloe vera applied to burns will help the healing process.

Egg whites slightly beaten and applied to first- and second-degree burns will take out the pain at once.

In the hospital in Turkey, when a person was badly burned, we made a quart of icy cold black tea and poured it over the burn again and again. They healed very quickly.

For minor burns, running icy cold water continuously for several minutes will be so effective, no other treatment is necessary. If serious burns are involved, begin cold water therapy and call for medical help at once.

~ Bursitis ~

The homeopathic remedy that may help with bursitis is called *Arsenicum metallicum.*

To help bursitis, take 2 parts magnesium and 1 part calcium.

See a chiropractor.

~ Calluses ~

*see also Corns

Lemon and castor oil have been used with great success for corns and calluses. Take a piece of lemon and tie it over the corns overnight. Every night take a new piece of lemon and repeat.

Rub peppermint oil on calluses to help heal them.

When you have very sensitive corns on your feet, take the homeopathic remedy *Ranunculus bulbosus* (buttercup).

Soak your feet in warm water for about 15 minutes. Then cut a small piece of lemon peel and place the inside of it against your corn, tying it on, and let it stay there all night. Do this for several nights and the corn should lift out.

Soak feet in very warm water for five minutes or so, then buff with pumice to remove dead skin.

– Cancer –

Garlic has been found to block the formation of colon cancer and may prevent many other cancers.

Concord grape juice may help combat cancer in the following way: Every morning for six weeks, drink 1 quart of concord grape juice from the time you wake up until noon, with no other food during that time. After noon, begin eating normally. You should emphasize almonds, asparagus, and other fruits and vegetables and have no heavy protein after 2 p.m. This is used in Europe with outstanding results.

Cabbage has been called the medicine of the poor and is extremely valuable for its healing qualities. Research indicates that cabbage contains ingredients which prevent cancer, making it an important addition to any diet.

Beets have an anti-carcinogenic hormone.

Asparagus contains substances that assist the body in normal cell formation. Asparagus contains a great deal of iodine and may be helpful in preventing cancer and other cell-destroying diseases. It is especially helpful with tumors.

In the old country, dried boiled orange peelings were used for cancer patients having pain, particularly if the cancer was in the mouth or the tongue.

The following list of fruits and vegetables all contain carotenoids that are antioxidants protecting against cancer:

> apricots
> cantaloupe
> carrots
> citrus fruits
> kale
> parsley
> spinach
> sweet potatoes
> turnip greens
> winter squash
> yams

Broccoli, cucumber, eggplant, pepper, and tomatoes all have plant steroids that block estrogen promotion in breast cancer.

Tomatoes and red grapefruit have "Lycopines," the active chemical ingredients in food which are antioxidants, also protecting against cancer.

Green tea and berries contain catachins as the active chemical ingredients in food which are antioxidants, protecting against cancer.

～ Candida Albicans ～

*see also Irritable Bowel Syndrome

Rosemary is thought to encourage the immune system and is thought to improve candida conditions.

Savory is antibacterial, antifungal, and antiviral, and has been used to treat staph and candida.

Candida albicans looks like an algae in the ocean. It settles in the mucosal surface of the intestine and will not bother us when kept in check. The early symptoms of candiasis area:

- frequent headaches
- dizziness
- poor digestion
- fatigue
- nausea
- white coating on the tongue and nearly all types of allergic reactions
- yeast infections
- blurred vision
- rectal itch
- rashes

Two time-tested herb formulas are Kantita and Foon Goos #2.

What makes candida albicans so poisonous? Candida is diagnosed when there is an abnormally high fungus in the intestinal tract. It reaches the fatal stage when the toxins enter the blood stream and start biting the hypothalamus, causing all types of mental aberrations from suicidal depression to homicidal attacks. This is a toxic brain poisoning and not an emotional problem. Not everyone's symptoms are the same. In short, the waste of the fungus attacks the nervous system. Candida also inhibits biotin, inositol, and methionine from being manufactured and distributed.

~ Carpal Tunnel Syndrome ~

Vitamins B_{12}, B_6, calcium and magnesium, and zinc will all help to combat carpal tunnel syndrome.

Here is what you can do:
First: Rub palms upward ten times (starting with pinky finger)

FIRST EXERCISE

Then: In the order shown, rotate wrist while
       holding point shown.

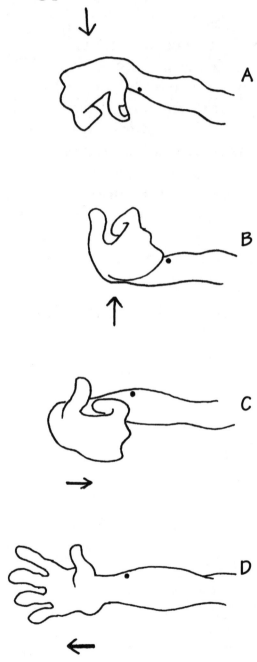

Carpal tunnel syndrome is caused by compression of the median nerve in between the tendons of the forearm muscles by a shrinking of the circular wrist ligament that holds everything together. This compressed nerve causes radiating pain in the palm of the hand and wrist, especially when the underside of the wrist is forcefully tapped with an index finger or a reflex hammer.

Treatment includes B_6 at 75 mg t.i.d., zinc at 50 mg t.i.d.

~ Cataracts ~

*see also Eye Problems

The following is a treatment for cataracts in the eyes: take fresh coconut juice and with an eye dropper, apply as much as the eye can hold. Apply hot wet cloths for about 10 minutes while lying down. Several treatments are needed.

Farmers use horseradish for cataracts and inflammation of the eyes. The root is grated and eaten raw, or a broth is made.

Dr. Alex Duarte has researched into the nutrients involved in cataract development. His approach is claimed to be 80% effective in combating senile cataracts. Dr. Duarte takes vitamin C, cystein, and methionine. These two amino acids are known to be of a sulphur-rich family. Eggs, garlic, beans, and onions are rich in these amino acids. The dosage for methionine supplementation is 200–1000 mg daily between meals.

— Celiac Disease —

Banana is a Godsend in celiac. Children are so limited with their food intake, but banana goes well and by-and-by corrects the altered intestinal functions.

There may be a selenium deficiency in people with celiac.

Apple can be given in celiac but must be first finely grated.

Celiac disease (gluten enteropathy, nontropical sprue) is perhaps the most underrated disease in America today. Celiac disease is characterized by a loss of villi (finger-like projections) from the small intestines and a scarring of the supporting tissue which effectively reduces the absorptive surface by 70%. Classically, celiac disease is caused by a wheat gluten sensitivity, thus "gluten free diets." If this change was limited to wheat only, it would be of small consequence because it is easily recognized; however, cow's milk, albumen, and soy protein will cause these same physical changes in the gut including loss of villi and scarring of supportive tissue of the small intestine progressing to the point where by age 45–50 years, 90% of the intestine can be damaged resulting in a significant reduction of absorptive surface. The result is poor assimilation of nutrients which are the raw materials for tissue repair, growth, and maintenance of the immune system.

Celiac disease is, therefore, the basic cause of many diseases including diabetes (e.g., malabsorption of chromium and vanadium), cancer (e.g., malabsorption of zinc, vitamin A, and selenium), and muscular dystrophy and cystic fibrosis (e.g., malabsorption of selenium in the pregnant mother resulting in damage to the fetus).

Diagnosis and treatment of celiac disease includes using the pulse test for allergies (e.g., whole wheat is great unless you're allergic to it!), especially wheat, cow's milk, and soy products, and eliminating and/or rotating the offending allergen. It takes 90 days to repair the injured gut, which means there is great hope if you take the effort to see if, in fact, you are sensitive to wheat, cow's milk, or soy.

~ Cellulite ~

Eggplant is very useful for cellulite. It first has to be sliced and placed in slightly salted water for about 20 minutes or more. This will remove the bitterness. The skin is extremely helpful. Peel the eggplant one half inch thick. Boil the peelings until done. Season with kelp or dulse. This is excellent for cellulite.

Sage, when added to bathwater is absorbed through the skin and fights fatty deposits from the inside out. You may also use sage oil.

~ **Cholesterol** ~

Alfalfa sprouts will help rid the body of excess cholesterol, only if taken in small quantities.

An apple a day can help lower cholesterol.

Garlic, onions, leek, and chives inhibit cholesterol synthesis and protect against carcinogens. The active food component is called "allylic sulfides."

When taken in capsules, cayenne may help reduce cholesterol buildup.

Increase your fruit, niacin, and vitamin C to help lower your cholesterol level.

Try the herbal product "Kolester."

Taurine is an amino acid that works exceptionally well in helping to lower high cholesterol levels and high blood pressure. Studies also show that it seems able to help control heart rhythm irregularities. Most importantly, taurine has been proven to help in the treatment of epilepsy. At the Atkins Center, we have been able to get at least 40 percent of patients with seizure disorder off their medications.

~ **Circulation Problems** ~

*see also Angina, Arteries, Heart Disease
Fennel is a circulatory stimulant.

Ginger is an excellent stimulant for both the circulatory system and the immune system.

Poor circulation can be caused by cardiovascular disease, low thyroid, and vitamin E deficiency. Symptoms include cold hands and feet and numb tingling fingers and toes.

For help with circulation problems, try rosemary, lily of the valley, *Convallaria majalis* (homeopathic), and ginseng.

Circu Flow is an herbal product.

~ Colds ~

For an excellent natural cold remedy, combine bay leaves with cinnamon, sage, and cloves, and boil them in apple juice.

Lemon balm, garlic, or cayenne pepper appear to deter colds and flu when taken at the onset of the illness.

Myrrh tincture relieves infectious ailments like colds.

For relief of a head cold, inhale warm vapors of myrtle in boiled water.

Eating currants or kale helps build resistance to colds.

Celery increases the appetite, and is good in curing mucous conditions. Therefore it is used for colds and coughs.

~ Cold Sores ~

Take two carrots finely grated. Place them

between two layers of a cotton cloth and apply to the sores. Change every two hours.

Lysine helps block the reproduction of the herpes virus. Some natural sources of lysine are brewer's yeast, milk, meat, and soybeans.

Foods to avoid if you suffer from cold sores are chocolate, gelatin, and nuts.

To help relieve canker sores, apply a wet, black tea bag to the area.

Olive leaf compound is excellent.

~ Colic ~

Fennel has been used as a medicine to help relieve colic conditions. Add one teaspoon fennel seeds to one cup water. Bring to a boil and simmer for about ten minutes. Strain and give children only one teaspoon in water.

Gentian is a fabulous tonic for colic. Make a tea of it, and give one teaspoon in a warm cup of water to children.

Caraway and anise mixed together are great for colic. Make a tea.

Yam has also been called "colic root" for its soothing properties in colic conditions.

Allspice has been known to relieve colic.

Cinnamon is not only a sweet spice, but it also has been used for colic.

Diluted dill tea is very helpful in calming colic conditions.

Cardamom warms and stimulates the body and is used for colic.

Peppermint is another helper in colic conditions.

A tea made from fenugreek will help colitis.

～ **Colon Problems** ～

Pears, rhubarb, and rutabagas are great colon cleansers.

When the abdomen is distended and bloated, try extra calcium. When it is distended without nausea, try ½ teaspoon of nutmeg in hot water. If you are suffering from abdominal tenderness, either linden flower tea internally, or H-12 (12 herb solution) externally on the navel may help.

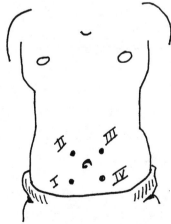

Press number I for stomach. Press number II for duodenum. Press number III for small intestine. Wherever it is sore, hold the spot to heal the correspondent organ.

~ Constipation ~

Oranges and thyme are good digestive tonics, and help in constipation.

Eat plenty of prunes and apples when you feel constipated.

To overcome hardened bowel movements, simmer one teaspoon of dill seed in one cup of boiling water, strain, and eat the hot seeds on bread. Drink the remaining tea for improvement of digestive processes.

Fennel, sesame seeds, or flaxseeds help relieve constipation.

Another remedy for constipation is to buy psyllium seeds and to crush them. Add a little water and prepare a mash to take before bedtime as needed. Add high fiber oat bran for especially stubborn cases.

~ Corns ~

*see also Calluses
To relieve the pain of corns, soak in Epsom salts and never wear tight shoes.

Massage your feet.

~ Cough ~

*see also Bronchial Trouble,
 Bronchitis, Lung, Respiratory
For a nagging cough or a tickling larynx, sip on red onion soup. The following soup recipe is excel-

lent: Take several red onions and break them up. Include the papery skin. Simmer in water for about 20 minutes and strain. Sip on a little of this broth every hour until relief is obtained.

Eating oranges helps relieve thick mucous-type coughing and is thought to relieve and prevent colds. Active ingredient: *limonoids.*

For a very dry cough, cut up onions, boil in vinegar for 15 minutes and add honey. Take one teaspoon every hour. Active ingredient: *allylic sulfide.*

For coughs due to colds, boil one pint of water, add a pinch of cayenne, a slice of lemon, two tablespoons of honey, and one ounce of shredded slippery elm. Allow to stand ½ hour then strain. Take frequently in small doses.

For whooping cough, take one teaspoon of wild cherry bark 3 times daily.

Another remedy for whooping cough is to take one tablespoon of sage in a pint of water and take one teaspoon five times a day.

Cloves and celery are both very useful in coughs. *Phenolic acid* is the active ingredient.

A tea made from the leaves of borage has been found to reduce dry rasping coughs.

Fennel is great for chronic coughs, and other respiratory complaints.

Cinnamon has been found to be helpful for asthma, wheezing, and coughing.

Whooping Cough:
Use homeopathic *Drosera rotundifolia* for whooping cough. ⤸

⁓ Crohn's Disease ⁓

Crohn's disease patients have a protozoan infection. Take Protozoa Kit.

Also, eat food rich in vitamin E.

Olive leaves will help to counteract both protozoa and viroid infections. ⤸

⁓ Curved Spine ⁓

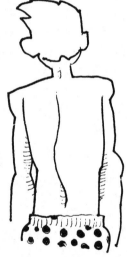

Sleeping on an oat straw mattress is thought to heal the bones and to straighten out a curved spine. The curse of a curved spine goes way back to your ancestors, as T.B. residue. This is carried on to your life. No problem! Ask for homeopathic "T.B. Residue." It will take quite a while to correct it.

Hammertoe also is "T.B. residue." ⤸

– Cuts –

For a paper cut on the finger, wet the finger and dip it into powdered cloves. The pain quickly disappears because of the clove's anesthetic effect on the skin.

A mixture of apple juice and olive oil has been used as an antiseptic for cuts and abrasions.

– Cysts –

The homeopathic remedy for cysts is "Epigea Homae" (trailing arbutus).

Free your body from parasites, chemicals, and viral infections. Only then can your body fight the cysts that have formed.

See other books.

– Dandruff –

Boil a handful of willow leaves, strain and wash your hair and scalp in it. Put a little of the tea aside and dampen the scalp every day a little.

Lack of B vitamins can result in dandruff.

– Depression –

Oranges are useful when fighting depression.

Borage as a tea is helpful for grief, anxiety, and depression.

To help through soothing times, teas made from both anise and thyme are soothing.

Oats can be helpful in our quest for health and well being. They are thought to relieve depression and nervous disorders.

Rosemary is uplifting, energizing, and therefore helpful in depression cases.

Clove tea can also be used for depression. It is said that the aroma of clove tea will create a feeling of protection and courage.

Taking extra pantothenic acid and vitamin B_6 may help depression.

Garlic has helped people who feel discouraged and who have negative thoughts. Burn the garlic skin slowly on an incense burner to help right away. It is a mild tranquilizer.

Clove concentrate can help because it has a soothing, slightly sedative effect on the body. To make it, bruise a handful of cloves, steep in boiling water, then simmer for a few minutes. Do not allow the water to be reduced too much or it will be too strong. One teaspoon of this mixture added to one cup of hot water will help tremendously.

Black snake root was chewed by the Indians to calm the nerves and to alleviate depression.

Lemon balm and daisy tea has a calming effect on the body. Therefore it is wonderful for depression.

Confusion:

To help a confused person, have them drink ginger tea, about ½ cup twice a day. ⮑

– **Dermatitis** –

*see also Eczema, Skin

Taking an oatmeal bath has been a home remedy for dermatitis for decades.

When you have sore and raw spots on the feet, use red onion to eat. Combined with vinegar, it will remove blemishes. In homeopathy it is called *Allium cepa.* ⮑

– **Diabetes** –

*see also Hypoglycemia

See your physician before treating yourself for diabetes.

For diabetes, drink two cups of dwarf leaf tea a day.

Devil's claw in capsules may help diabetes.

Drink either blueberry leaf tea, blackberry leaf tea, or oat straw tea for diabetes. Boil the leaves and drink four cups daily.

White figs as compresses over the throat have been useful in diabetes.

The avocado is a fat and protein supplier and is great food for the diabetic. Combine avocado with agar-agar (dry), lime juice, and raw rolled oats. Drink plenty of distilled water between meals.

Hypoglycemia and diabetes sufferers may be deficient in chromium.

Garlic helps regulate blood sugar levels and is known to be beneficial in cases of adult onset diabetes.

The following minerals and vitamins should be included in the diabetic's diet:

> chromium
> inositol
> vitamin C
> magnesium
> garlic
> niacin
> anthocyanic acid (blueberry extract)
> zinc
> vitamin B_6
> acidophilus

People with diabetes or any kind of reduced feeling in their feet should never treat themselves. Due to the tiny blood vessels being affected by diabetes, they have a tendency for wounds that do not heal and for increased infections.

All people with pancreas trouble should consider clearing the pancreas from flukes. I use a homeopathic formula called Pancreatic Flukes.

～ Diarrhea ～

To relieve diarrhea, make a tea from the green leaves of sunflower, and drink several cups.

Strained carrots, cinnamon, apples, or rice gruel are all excellent in relieving diarrhea.

Cardamom warms and stimulates the body and is used for diarrhea.

Barley is an excellent food for children suffering from diarrhea or other inflammation of the bowels.

Cayenne is especially helpful for diarrhea and cramps.

Blackberries are colon food and are great for diarrhea.

The apple agrees with most people. Raw and finely grated, apples will stop your children's diarrhea.

Iceberg lettuce water is used in cases of diarrhea.

Nutmeg will help relieve diarrhea.

～ Digestion ～

*see also Flatulence, Gas, Intestinal Difficulties

Garlic is useful in digestive disorders such as gastroenteritis and dysentery.

Nutmeg aids digestive problems.

Cardamom is commonly used to treat indigestion and gas. It warms and stimulates the body.

Lettuce, like spinach, is rich in vitamins A, B, C, and E. It stimulates the smooth operation of the digestive tract and adds needed bulk to the diet.

Dill tea helps relieve gas, indigestion, and cramps. To make dill tea, use one teaspoon dill seeds to eight ounces cold water and bring to a boil. Simmer for ten minutes. Drink before or with a meal.

Lemon balm helps indigestion, especially during worry or anxiety. It is antibacterial and antiviral in nature, probably because it contains tannins.

Peppermint is well known to help indigestion, intestinal spasms, gas, and other similar conditions, particularly in children. Peppermint leaves in cottage cheese taste good and help digestion.

Bay leaf is a digestive aid and stimulates the appetite.

Cabbage and kale are helpful for digestive problems because they induce protective enzymes.

Fennel in food will help digestion greatly. Too much stomach acidity can be regulated by taking one cup of fennel tea. Fennel expels mucus and relieves cramps, gas, and indigestion. Chewing fennel seeds relieves hunger and eases digestion. It is delicious and naturally sweet.

Cinnamon can be used as an aid to digestive processes and alleviates indigestion, cramps, and gas.

Tomatoes will help digest protein, but do not eat the part where the stem attaches to the tomato.

Artichokes help improve weak digestion.

Sage improves digestive function and helps the body digest protein.

Arrowroot is very easily digestible, creating no gastric upset. It forms a nourishing diet. People suffering from bacillary dysentery and gastric upset would find it most suitable. Take a teaspoonful of arrowroot, make a smooth paste with cold milk or water, stir well, and boil. Add a little lime juice just before taking it.

Ginger has been used for digestive disorders.

Oranges are used as a digestive remedy, aiding in the treatment of constipation.

Thyme is a digestive tonic, improving sluggish digestion. It has been used for gastric problems such as colic, indigestion, and gas.

Alfalfa seeds are loaded with vitamin C and vitamin K. Alfalfa contains many trace minerals that improve digestion.

Caraway is very much like anise, and when mixed with anise, it is twice as good. It is antispasmodic, and subsides gastric distention. It is a digestive aid, and is used to prevent cramping when added to laxative formula.

Some people cannot digest bananas. After eating bananas, chew a few cinnamon seeds and the indigestion caused by bananas will be alleviated.

Papaya has been used for protein digestion.

Mustard, horseradish, and radishes are known to raise vital life forces and is helpful in digestion, because it makes protective digestive enzymes.

Coriander is a digestive tonic and is a mild sedative. It is helpful for gas and indigestion.

Celery aids in protein digestion. It increases appetite, is good in curing mucus, and therefore is used in gastric trouble.

Marjoram has been used for gastrointestinal difficulties.

Citrus fruit and bell peppers both make protective enzymes that aid in digestion.

For slow digestion, take Homeopathic Lycopodium (club moss).

~ **Diuretic** ~

Cucumber satisfies thirst, and it is a very good diuretic.

Lack of potassium is known to cause leg cramps, especially at night. Before you take potassium pills, ask yourself how much fruit you are eating. Because of the potassium content, bananas can also balance excess water in the system and are good to relieve waterlogged tissues.

Juniper berries are a gentle stimulant and diuretic.

Asparagus is a wonderful diuretic. It is cooling, soothing, and a tremendous addition to any diet, especially when tumors are present.

For a diuretic, take equal parts of caraway, fennel, and anise (about one teaspoon of each) and add to one pint of water. Bring to a boil and simmer for fifteen minutes. Drink this amount twice a day.

– Diverticulosis –

The cause of diverticulosis is a protozoan infection.

To help with diverticulosis, eat no wheat, and drink fennel tea to relieve bloatedness.

– Dropsy –

For dropsy, take broom tops in capsules or as a tea.

Potato peelings are helpful with dropsy. Boil the peelings and drink six ounces twice a day.

For dropsy, elder flower tea, two cups a day, will help.

Horseradish in apple juice, one half cup, three times a day will help dropsy. Take one half gallon apple cider plus a handful of parsley (crushed), a handful of horseradish (crushed), and a tablespoon of juniper berries combined, and let stand for 24 hours in a warm place. Drink a half glass three times a day before meals.

~ **Drug Residue** ~

Make a dish with lima beans, bell peppers, and sweet potato to combat drug residue.

For heroin deposits, make chaparral tea, two cups a day or in capsules.

Tobacco leaf tea added to bath water will help combat drug residue.

To quit a morphine habit, eat oats, and celery root, called "celeriac."

Chromium and vanadium is missing in the brain.

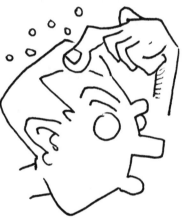

~ **Earache** ~

For an earache, take a cotton ball, soak it in a little bit of mineral oil, and sprinkle fresh ground pepper on it. Place it over the ear, not directly in the ear canal, and secure with a Band-Aid.

Cayenne is indicated when the ears are stinging or burning, when there is swelling behind the ears, or for Eustachian tube difficulties. If the ears are burning, drink cayenne in a little hot water. If there is a swelling behind the ear, put cayenne in a little water and rub on the back of the ear.

Eating grapefruit is helpful if you have ringing in the ears or other head noises. Try eating a piece of grapefruit if you have pain in the temporal region.

For ear problems such as recurring ear infection or ringing in the ear, cut a yellow onion in half and rub on the back of the ear.

For inner ear trouble, take one handful of horsetail, boil, and strain. Add to your bath. Soak for twenty minutes.

For stinging or shooting pain in the ear, use violet leaf tea.

For swelling behind the ear, take a cloth and moisten it, sprinkle with freshly ground pepper and apply.

For a swollen gland near the ear, take ground flax seed, mix it with salt, put between layers of cloth, and apply.

For an earache, drop a little garlic oil into the ear. Leave it for only ten minutes and then remove it with some cotton. For flu or colds, take one teaspoon of the oil every hour. To prepare garlic oil, take one half pound of peeled and crushed garlic cloves. Put in a jar and cover with olive oil. Close tightly and shake a few times each day for three days, storing in a warm place. Strain through a clean cotton cloth. Store this garlic oil in a cool place.

Chamomile tea can be used for ringing in the ears. ⟿

~ **Eczema** ~

*see also Dermatitis, Skin
Flax seed contains a remarkable healing oil which can be used externally or internally. Flax oil is useful for eczema.

If you suffer from eczema with ulceration, drink three cups of clove water a day.

The oil extracted from the seeds of borage is available in capsules and is applied to the skin for eczema and other rashes or dry skin. ⟿

~ **Emotional** ~

*see also Grief
For emotional sensitivity, take thuja tea, or *Thuja occidentalis* homeopathic.

For emotional upset, drink one cup of Meadow Sweet tea, sweetened with honey.

For other types of emotional trouble, take homeopathic *Ignatia amara* (St. Ignatius' bean). ⟿

~ **Emphysema** ~

*see also Bronchial Trouble,
  Cough, Lung, Respiratory
For emphysema, take Sound Breath and Foon Goos, and more vitamins C and E. ⟿

~ Exhaustion ~

For exhaustion, take dried whey, one table-spoon, two times daily.

Also take thyme tea for exhaustion.

~ Eye Problems ~

*see also Cataracts, Pinkeye

Cardamom is an eye and brain food.

Bell pepper is good for the eyes.

If you have the sensation of gauze before your eyes, take linden flower tea, two cups a day.

To strengthen the eyes, make angelica root tea, one half cup twice a day with maple syrup.

To help correct loss of eyesight because of diabetes, take a zinc supplement, and eat Hungarian paprika daily.

To help with loss of eyesight because of tobacco, take more vitamins B_{12}, and folic acid daily.

If you have a twitching eyelid, drink elder flower tea, and vitamin B_6.

White beans are good for the eyes.

If you have retina bleeding, take the following:

vitamin C
rutin
vitamin B_1

bioflavonoids
Hungarian paprika
raw potato compresses

Sunflower seeds are great for the eyes. They are very helpful for eyestrain and sensitivity to light. Nibble about a half a cup of seeds daily.

If your eye aches, take calcium fluoride.

If you suffer from an atrophy of the optic nerve, bathe in tobacco water.

For a burning sensation in your eye, take eyebright tea, two cups daily, and also vitamins A and B_{12}.

For conjunctivitis, place a raw potato on the eye.

Carrots are of great use for health, but should not be used in excess. Drink the juice slowly. They help prevent night blindness.

Fennel can be used as an eyewash. Make a tea of it, strain, and then bathe your eyes with it. It has been used throughout history to improve eyesight.

The homeopathic remedies for eye problems are Argentum Nitrate and Silver Nitrate.

For sties on the eye, make a poultice of black tea, place moist over the eye, and bandage it overnight.

If your eyes water all the time, take Homeopathic Euphrasia and Eyebright.

Rosemary has been used with great success to help the eyesight.

Eye treatment:

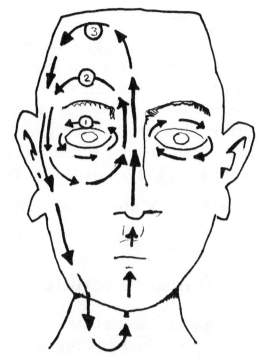

Massage every day.

~ Fallout ~

*see also Radiation

To treat fallout, eat cloves with vitamin C, and/or willow leaf tea, about two cups daily.

Cinnamon removes fallout. Toast one side of bread very brown. Butter it and put cinnamon on it. If you like, also put some brown sugar on it. This counteracts radiation.

To remove radioactive fallout, add one pound of baking soda and one half pound of salt to your bath.

Seaweed and miso soup have a neutralizing effect in radiation overdose.

A formula to counteract radioactive fallout is as follows: Take one glass of cranberry juice, one quarter teaspoon cinnamon, one quarter teaspoon powdered clove, and one quarter teaspoon cream of tartar. This drink is very delicious and helpful. Also willow leaves have been found to help remove all symptoms of this illness.

A willow leaf bath for children and weak adults will help for fallout.

– Female Trouble –

*see also Menopause, Menstrual, PMS
Thyme has been used historically for female disorders, and it seems to have an affinity to the uterus. It also can be used to relieve menstrual pain and restore balance during abnormal absence of menstrual periods.

Yams seem to be helpful to menopausal women.

Okra is a general tonic for the body and is useful in cases of heavy menstrual bleeding.

Black cohosh, sarsaparilla, vitamin B₁, and licorice tea have all been useful for PMS.

Sage contains natural estrogen.

The following recipe is helpful for lumps in the ovaries: Take two parts of calendula, one part of plantain, and one part of yarrow. Make a tea, and drink one quart of it daily for four weeks.

To help with the circulation to the uterus, make tansy tea, and drink one half cup two times daily.

For cramping in the uterus, drink cramp bark tea, one half cup, two times daily.

If the uterus is enlarged, drink yarrow tea.

Apply ice to the nipples to stop uterine bleeding.

Oats are rich in silicon. They stimulate sweating and are helpful for estrogen deficiency.

Fig leaves help strengthen the lining of the uterus.

To promote menstrual flow, drink motherwort tea.

For a scanty menstrual flow, drink thyme tea.

For trouble with no menstrual flow, drink yarrow tea, two cups daily.

Clotting will stop if you drink shepherd's purse, two cups daily.

If your menstruation is disturbed because of emotional upset, take Homeopathic Tiger Lily.

Okra helps to regulate female bleeding.

Fennel tea is helpful to the reproductive system. It is an old folk remedy to regulate difficult and irregular menstrual periods. It has a hormonal-like action that reduces the effect of PMS and menopausal symptoms. Use fennel tea up to three times daily before and during your period.

Endometriosis:

Take Kantita and Foon Goos #2, and thyme tea for endometriosis. ⬎

– Fever –

For fever in children, give them diluted yellow jasmine tea, Homeopathic Gelsemium, and Homeopathic Echinacea.

For intermittent fever, take holly tea.

To reduce fever, take pleurisy root.

For tic fever, take three tablets of chaparral, three times daily for one month.

Gentian alleviates fevers, cools the body, and maintains digestive functions during a fever to prevent stagnation of food.

As a tea for fever, use equal parts of cardamom and clovers.

Dried apple peelings made into a tea will strengthen muscles, weakness, and is good in rheumatic fever.

Hot lemon juice with honey is good for fevers.

Coriander as a tea can relieve fever.

Marjoram tea is a mild tonic which aids fever situations.

Make willow bark tea, and sip slowly for fevers. ⬎

~ Fibromyalgia ~

Add malic acid (from apples) and 100 mg manganese and 800 mg magnesium.

The presence of protozoa in the tissue can also cause fibromyalgia. Take the Protozoa Kit.

No wheat.

~ Flatulence ~

*see also Digestion, Gas, Intestinal Difficulties
Either anise or lemon balm can be used to relieve flatulence.

~ Flu ~

Sip on red onion soup if you feel an oncoming flu.

Grapefruit is a lime supplier and is good for the flu.

Oranges have vitamin C for flu prevention.

Cayenne helps prevent colds and flu.

An ordinary back rub can activate your immune system to help you beat the flu quickly.

Onion Soup for Flu:
Cut one large yellow onion in small pieces. Cover it up with 2 quarts water. Simmer for a half hour. Strain, and add a little honey to taste. Drink 2 cups every two hours until flu is gone.

Garlic and onion (allylic sulfides) stimulate production of a detoxifying enzyme.

- Fluid Retention -

*see also Bloated Condition,
  Water-Logged Tissues
Cabbage has been used with great success for fluid retention.

See a physician for heart trouble and for kidney trouble.

- Food Poisoning -

To combat food poisoning, take two teaspoons of apple cider vinegar in seven ounces of warm water and sip slowly. For children, add honey.

Gentian is helpful for food poisoning.

For botulism, take six parts of pokeroot, and three parts of sarsaparilla, and make a strong tea. Give one tablespoon every half hour.

Nutmeg aids food poisoning as well.

Ginger tea with honey.

- Foot Problems -

Apply mashed, ripe tomatoes to the sole of your painful feet, or just apply a few slices. Bandage these to your soles and leave on all night. The next morning, all soreness should be gone from your feet.

The homeopathic remedy for sore and raw feet is Allium Cepa (red onion).

Soak tired feet in warm water with two tablespoons of Epsom salts.

For feet that smell, soak them in ordinary black tea for ten or fifteen minutes, three times a week. The components in the tea help close pores and stop the sweating.

Athlete's Foot:
Quaw bark tincture applied externally will help athlete's foot.

- Forgetfulness -

*see also Brain, Memory
The homeopathic remedy for forgetfulness is Carbonate of Ammonia.

- Gallbladder Trouble -

Make pumpkin seed tea by taking one teaspoon of ground pumpkin seeds, pour one cup of hot water over them, and let it steep for a few minutes. Drink two cups of tea daily for gallbladder help.

Radishes in small amounts promote bile flow.

Artichokes increase the flow of bile.

For chronic gall bladder trouble, obstruction, or pain in the bladder, take Homeopathic Chelidonium.

The whole apple is balm to the gallbladder.

Artichokes bring clear urine and increase flow of bile.

Pumpkin seed tea is great for gallbladder troubles. Take one heaping teaspoon of ground pumpkin seeds. Put seven ounces of hot water over it and drink slowly. Two cups a day are needed to help the gallbladder.

Two teaspoons of lemon juice before each meal will strengthen the gallbladder.

Horseradish raw or dried will aid the gallbladder.

~ Gallstones ~

The following recipe will help combat gallstones:

First Day:

8 am	1 glass (8 oz) apple juice
10 am	2 glasses (16 oz) apple juice
12 pm	2 glasses (16 oz) apple juice
2 pm	2 glasses (16 oz) apple juice
4 pm	2 glasses (16 oz) apple juice
6 pm	2 glasses (16 oz) apple juice

The apple juice should be natural, without chemicals. No food is to be taken this day.

Second Day:

Follow the same procedure as the first day. No food this day either. At bedtime drink four ounces of olive oil. You may wash the olive oil down with hot lemon juice. Go to bed at once.

Another remedy for gallstones is to take two tablespoons of grated black radish blended with one tablespoon olive oil. Take twenty minutes before meals for gallstones.

The homeopathic remedy for gallstones is Chionoutus (fringe tea).

~ Gas ~

*see also Digestion, Flatulence, Intestinal Difficulties

Allspice has been known to relieve gas.

For stomach gas, take one teaspoon of CERTO and add it to one half glass of apple juice, and drink as needed.

~ Gastrointestinal Difficulties ~

*see Digestion

~ Germicide ~

Cinnamon is a natural germicide.

Olive Leaf compound is also a natural helper.

~ Glandular Problems ~

Chicken, chick peas, sweet potatoes, yams, sesame seeds, sunflower seeds, and avocado served without oil or butter are all gland foods.

A slice of tomato on glandular swelling removes it quickly.

Green tomatoes in very small amounts are a gland stimulant. Always remove the core and the stem. Make a deep insertion. The stem part is poisonous.

Boil plantain leaves and mix with salt. Use it as a compress for swollen glands.

Marjoram is great for glandular problems.

Plantain oil can be applied to neutralize poisons.

Dandelion root stimulates the glands.

Alfalfa seed tea nourishes the glands.

Yucca is similar to cortisone and is an adrenal gland food.

Mullein leaf tea if good for the glandular system. Drink two cups daily.

Sabal serrulata (saw palmetto) homeopathic or saw palmetto tincture, are good to strengthen glandular tissue.

When there is a burning or cutting feeling in the glands that gets worse at night, try horseradish.

Used as a poultice of hot milk and crushed seeds, fenugreek relieves swollen glands.

Use sage for glandular weakness and bloated conditions.

– Gout –

*see also Stone and Gout

Sour cherries are a good remedy for gout by eating one small dish of sour cherries every morning for three weeks. Eat cherries morning and night for hypochondria.

Drink lots of fluids, at least two quarts daily.

Gout is actually a form of arthritis, when there is too much uric acid in the blood. To lower uric acid, take activated charcoal by mouth, one half teaspoon to one teaspoon four times daily.

Apple cider vinegar, honey, and water together may be used to "balance" the body. This combination is beneficial for people with gout.

Combine avocado with agar-agar (dry), lime juice, and raw rolled oats. Drink plenty of distilled water between meals.

The homeopathic remedy for gout is Antimonium Crudum.

For the condition that is not quite yet gout, try Homeopathic Berberis.

– Grief –

*see also Emotional

Borage can be used for grief with great success.

– Gum Problems –

*see also Mouth, Teeth

If you have sore gums, make Hyssop tea and hold in the mouth several times daily.

Also Gingivitis Remedy.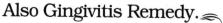

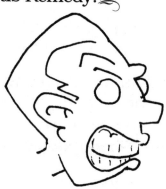

~ **Hair Loss** ~

Drink and rinse with cooled wormwood tea. Brew two tablespoons in one quart of water for twenty-five minutes. Cool before moistening the scalp.

Sarsaparilla tea or nettle tea are great drinks for combating hair loss.

Hair loss could be a sign of an underactive thyroid. Eat high protein with no sugar at all and plenty of yogurt.

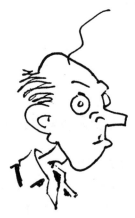

Cabbage is good for the hair.

Thyme tea is also found to be helpful to prevent or stop hair loss.

Emu-mu, 15 drops, once a day.

– Hangover –

Borage has been used for the relief of a hangover.

Thyme tea is helpful to detoxify from a hangover.

Cucumber reduces the intoxicating effect of alcohol.

Make fennel tea, strain, and put in the bath to detoxify the body and release toxic waste. This can also be helpful in a hangover situation.

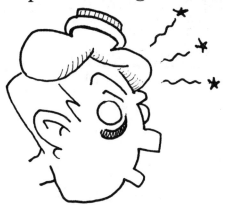

– Headaches –

*see also Migraines

Marjoram has been used extensively to reduce headaches.

The orange has been used for headaches with nausea or facial neuralgia, mostly right-sided. Peel the orange and eat one half of it at a time.

If you have a headache that originates at the back of the head, it could signal liver or gall-bladder trouble.

If your headache originates at the front of the head, it could mean kidney or bladder trouble.

Headaches that radiate from one point can be helped by drinking one cup of black tea.

For headaches with nausea, try Iris-Blue Flag Homeopathic.

Lady's slipper tea, lavender tea, and guarana tea can all help when a headache starts.

Lavender oil on the temples, NOT TO BE TAKEN INTERNALLY, can help ease a headache.

A simple but effective way to rid yourself of a headache is to tie a cloth snugly around the head.

For migraines, try vervain tea.

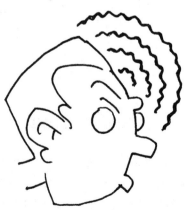

If you have a one-sided headache, take one half teaspoon of crushed allspice in juice twice daily.

Cabbage can be helpful if you have a headache.

The homeopathic remedies for headaches are Hyssop and Ferrum Picricum.

Cardamom warms and stimulates the body and can be used for headaches.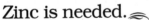

– Hearing Loss –

For deafness, try calendula or marigold.

Manganese will help prevent hearing loss.

Zinc is needed.

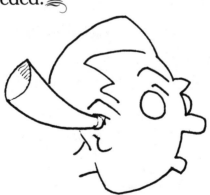

– Heartburn –

To avoid heartburn, take ginger just after you eat. Start with a small amount, and work up to the dosage that's just right for you.

– Heart Disease –

*see also Angina, Arteries, Circulation Problems

The following recipe is a heart-strengthener: Take two parts of cowslip and one part of lavender. Make a tea using one teaspoon per cup and drink two to three cups a day.

Blue malva flower tea is used for the heart valves. Drink one cup twice a day for six weeks.

Artichokes help keep the arteries smooth.

Parsley is a good food to keep arteries clear.

The homeopathic remedy for the heart is Aconite, derived from monkshood (?).

To strengthen the heart, use Homeopathic Arnica (leopard's bane). Use it after you have been overworked or overexerted.

If you have irregular palpitations, use Homeopathic Arsenicum.

Durum metallicum (gold) is a must in heart cases.

Bananas are high in potassium, which helps keep the heart in order.

Cabbage helps heart disorders.

Cayenne benefits the heart and prevents heart attacks and strokes. Cayenne taken in capsules helps treat cardiovascular disease by acting as a stimulant and reducing cholesterol build-up. It also normalizes circulation and can be used to stop bleeding.

Garlic is an excellent remedy for long-term cardiovascular difficulties. It reduces blood cholesterol, strengthens the arteries, and reduces the risk of further heart attacks in people who have already suffered one heart attack.

Parsley, carrots, winter squash, sweet potatoes, yams, cantaloupe, apricots, spinach, kale, turnip greens, and citrus fruits all have antioxidants that may help reduce accumulation of arterial plaque. They contain carotenoids.

Borage has been used historically to comfort the heart.

Apple tree bark is used to treat hardening of the arteries.

Vascular congestion can be treated by taking whey, a by-product of yogurt or cheese.

The homeopathic remedy for heart disease is Adonis (pheasant's eye).

Another homeopathic heart remedy is Convallaria Majalis (lily of the valley).

Heartbeat (irregular):
An irregular heartbeat (palpitations) can be the result of heart disease, food allergies, nutritional deficiencies, and/or hypoglycemia. Avoid caffeine, avoid offending food allergens, avoid sugar.

Most often a blockage in the heart muscle is the culprit.

See poisons as cadmium or nitrate.

Carnitine's greatest success is in the treatment of coronary insufficiency. It has also been shown to benefit cardiomyopathies and unstable heart rhythms, to decrease serum triglyceride and cholesterol levels, and to increase HDL (*International Journal of Cardiology*, vol. 5, 1984).

~ Heavy Metal Damage ~

Wheat sprouts will improve detoxification of tissue and protect against heavy metal damage in the body.

Time tested "Metaline" is terrific. (Herb formula. It was given in prayer.)

~ Hemorrhoids ~

*see also Piles

For general help with hemorrhoids, take vitamins B_6, calcium, chlorophyll, sesame seeds, and smart weed.

When you have painful and hot hemorrhoids, take ginger tea.

Collinsonia tea or capsules are helpful with hemorrhoids.

Use dandelion root tea, brewed fifteen minutes, to help with hemorrhoids. Drink two cups daily.

Oil a clove of garlic and insert it into the rectum each night for several nights in a row.

Make a poultice of cranberries to place externally over hemorrhoids.

Parsley is helpful for piles.

Eat three almonds daily to prevent and eliminate hemorrhoids.

Slice and dip a potato in oil to lubricate, and then insert it into the rectum for fast relief. Remember to pull it out after a while.

~ Herpes ~

Take buckbean tea, one cup daily, to help counteract herpes.

Club moss or Homeopathic Ranunculus will also help herpes as well.

A herpes infection is a tiny virus, making blisters and pain. Vitamin C, vitamin E, and zinc cream are recommended. In addition, eat foods rich in lysine, and a lysine supplement. (500 mg lysine once a day is sufficient.)

Olive leaf compound does an excellent job. In cases of retroviruses as found in HIV, hepatitis C, AIDS, and herpes infections, olive leaves do a superb job by inhibiting the growth with Elonolic Acid and Oleuropein, inside this holy plant.

~ Hiccups ~

A never-fail recipe for hiccups is to take an orange and cut it in half. Squeeze the juice from half the orange into a glass and drink it slowly. If needed, do the same with the other half.

Pineapple juice is a good source of vitamin C and can be used as a remedy for hiccups.

Anise tea is helpful for hiccups as well.

Massaging your earlobes will help ease hiccups.

To rid yourself of hiccups, eat a spoonful of sugar, suck on an ice cube, or yank on your tongue.

— High Blood Pressure —

*see Blood Pressure

— Hormones —

Yams are hormone food.

To boost a woman's hormone level, take one half cup of ground cashews, two tablespoons of rice polishings, two cups of water or apple juice, and blend in the blender. Add honey to taste.

— Human Papilloma Virus —

Use the PAP kit, and drink concord grape juice every day. You may also douche with concord grape juice as well.

After many years of working to help people the best I can, I feel that human papilloma virus is one of the most widespread viruses and must be treated. It can be devastating if not treated.

Papilloma becomes dangerous when it lodges in the female organs. It infects an estimated half million women every year. At the present time, 10 to 20 million women between the ages of 19 to 49 in this country alone are affected. World wide, however, cervical cancer is the second most common cancer in women and the most common and fatal cancer of women in developing countries. The importance of an annual Pap smear (which allows early detection in most cases) is highly advisable. Regular Pap smears are crucial in order to avoid drastic measures, especially since you can be infected with HPV and never have a symptom. Some symptoms are:

- tiredness
- cannot overcome Epstein-Barr virus
- genital warts (condyloma)
- dysplasia
- lack of concentration
- forgetfulness
- endometriosis
- abnormal Pap smear

A virus does not stay in one place. It migrates and goes to any part of the body. Therefore, total help is needed.

Again, use the PAP kit for this help.

− **Hyperactivity** −

*see also Attention Deficit Disorder

The cause of hyperactivity is a chemical poison in the nervous system.

Give homeopathic Chem-x to children with hyperactivity.

~ Hypochondria ~

Eat cherries morning and night for hypo-chondria.

~ Hypoglycemia ~

*see also Diabetes
Red beets are good for people with low blood sugar.

~ Immune System ~

To stimulate the immune system, take flaxseed and walnuts. They contain alpha linoleic acid.

~ Infection ~

Savory and basil are used to treat infections.

Boil cranberries and use the juice to fight infections.

Grate the skin of a grapefruit on a fine grater. Take one teaspoon and add the juice of one half grapefruit. Drink this three times daily to fight infection.

If you have an infection in the lung, boil onions, mash them and place them between two layers of cloth. Apply to chest for about two hours.

Make cabbage compresses for infections.

Take plenty of pantothenic acid when fighting an infection.

Virus infections take olive leaf compound.

Retrovirus infections take olive leaf compound.

~ Inflammation ~

Flaxseed, soy products, purslane, and walnuts all reduce inflammation and stimulate the immune system. They contain alpha linoleic acid.

Used as a poultice of hot milk and crushed seeds, fenugreek relieves inflammation.

Inflammation of the body may point to a protozoan infection. Take Protozoa Kit to help with inflammation.

~ Insomnia ~

*see also Sleeping Disorders

For insomnia due to worry, take prickly ash leaf tea, one cup at bedtime.

When an infant cannot sleep, make passion flower tea, and put two drops of tea to a cup of water.

Eating oranges helps calm the nerves and is useful for insomnia.

Thyme, dill, and lemon balm have been used for insomnia.

Warm a cup of milk and add one teaspoon of honey and drink before going to bed.

Always watch your heart. ⁓

~ Intestinal Difficulties ~

*see also Digestion
Eat yogurt for healthy intestines.

Check for parasites, especially protozoa. ⁓

~ Irritable Bowel Syndrome ~

*see also Candida Albicans
Borage and thyme have been used to treat irritable bowel syndrome. ⁓

~ Itching ~

Rub the inside of a banana peeling on the itching place. ⁓

~ Jaundice ~

Cucumber juice purifies the lymphatic system, cleans the blood, and relieves jaundice. Drink four or five cups of freshly pressed cucumber juice for this cleansing process.

Lime is used for yellow jaundice.

Artichokes and/or anise oil are good for jaundice.

Take Homeopathic Chionoutus (fringe tree) for jaundice.

See your physician. ⤵

~ **Jerking** ~

Take valerian root in capsules to relieve jerking.

Also take vitamin B_6 for jerking.

Jerking and Twitching:

Emu oil comes from the emu's thick back fat, yielding unsaturated, nontoxic, highly penetrating oil. Radiated with colors, it counteracts the poisons in the central nervous system such as nickel, lead, arsenic, cadmium, mercury, m.s.g., dioxin, aluminum, uranium, and nitrates. It stops jerking and twitching movements. Take 10 drops two times a day. ⤵

~ **Joints** ~

For stiff joints, the natural sodium in cucumber makes them more limber.

For joint cracking, give manganese.

Olive leaf compound is good. ⤵

~ **Kidney** ~

Make small cubes of watermelon and eat a small piece every fifteen minutes, all day long. This will relieve your kidney from mucus and accumulated poisons. Watermelon is for a sluggish kidney.

Horseradish boiled in apple juice gives copious urine if the kidney is blocked.

Juniper berries are extremely beneficial to the kidneys.

Parsley root has been used as a natural diuretic and to benefit kidney conditions.

Cut pears into small pieces and eat a piece every fifteen minutes all day to relieve the kidney.

Cabbage is very helpful with kidney disorders.

Celery has been used as a kidney cleanser for the removal of urinary stones. For kidney and bladder troubles, eat celery tops after each meal for five weeks.

Drink plenty of healthful cranberry juice every day to help your ailing kidneys.

Adzuki beans are for kidney trouble and swelling of the ankles.

Potato peelings are great for the kidneys.

Cinnamon is warming to the kidneys.

Cold pressed oils are needed to assimilate the proteins from vegetables. They are food to the kidney.

– Kidney Stones –

Asparagus is known to dissolve kidney stones.

Anise has historically been used to heal kidney stones. Put one tablespoon of anise in one quart of grape juice and simmer it for one half hour. Then drink seven ounces three times daily.

For kidney stones, drink one quart of parsley tea a day for three days. Then drink just two cups daily. Another option is to drink parsley tea for three days with no other food for these three days.

~ Lactation ~

Borage is good for lactation.

Fennel tea promotes lactation and can relieve colic in the nursing child.

Anise can enhance milk production in nursing mothers and relieve bloated conditions in the nursing child.

Anise will increase mother's milk also.

Caraway seeds will increase a nursing mother's milk. Take 1 teaspoon of caraway seeds and 8 ounces cold water. Bring to a boil and simmer for a few minutes. Drink several cups a day.

Dill tea will increase mother's milk.

~ Laryngitis ~

Thuja occidentalis homeopathic is good for chronic laryngitis.

Red onions are great for laryngitis.

Black bean juice is good for hoarseness and laryngitis. ⤳

— Lead Poisoning —

Ground ivy tea will help with lead poisoning. Drink two cups a day.

Lead is a toxic metal that is called by medical experts "one of the most common and persistent neurotoxins in the environment." It has been shown to cause damage at even very low levels. It is found in gasoline vapors, car exhaust, paint, hair dyes, tobacco smoke, and on the solder of tin cans. Every person is affected by it, but it is the children who are extremely vulnerable. They seem to absorb a much higher percentage of both inhaled and ingested lead. It causes a wide range of disorders including:

> lack of will power
> fatigue
> lack of abstract thinking
> allergies
> anemia
> headaches
> weakness
> hyperactivity in children
> brain disfunction

Lead causes a wide variety of problems in children and has been marked as one of the leading causes of children with behavioral and learning problems. Lead settles in the brain, nerves, bones, and the right kidney. There are ways to counteract the lead in our system:

The herb product "Metaline," which contains pumpkin seed, okra, rhubarb root, cayenne pepper, peppermint, and dulse.

Homeopathic "Plumbum."

~ Leg Cramps ~

Homeopathic *Arsenicum album* will help with leg cramps.

Lack of potassium can cause leg cramps.

Eat more fruit.

More calcium when left leg hurts.

More magnesium when right leg hurts.

~ Leukemia ~

Red beets are good for leukemia.

In all cases of leukemia, the tailbone should be checked and realigned.

This knowledge comes from Professor Dr. Brauchle. Professor Brauchle began using these non-medical methods in Dresden, Germany. In one wing of a 2,000-bed hospital, he worked with 25 patients per week, mostly children. Each week 25 patients would walk out perfectly healed. Not one died from leukemia.

Then and now, both science and medicine dismissed the results. They called these methods hocus pocus, magic, witchcraft, or some kind of hypnotherapy. It is none of these. We call it the healing power of God. Over 5,000 people who had leukemia used these methods and continued living. They call it something wonderful. ⌒

~ **Lice** ~

Mineral oil can get rid of lice. Pour warmed mineral oil over entire scalp. After 10 minutes, shampoo. Then use a fine-toothed comb to gather the suffocated lice. Repeat procedure every two days for ten days.

Thyme tea has been used as a skin antiseptic for lice. ⌒

~ **Liver** ~

White beans are helpful for the liver

Artichokes help to tone up the liver.

Allspice is a balm to the liver.

Apples can help stimulate the liver and digestive system.

Sage is also an excellent liver stimulant.

Cloves are beneficial to the liver when it is swollen and hard, damaged, or contains tumors.

Homeopathic Cheladonium is a remedy for the liver if it is swollen, painful, or if there is a bad odor.

Dandelion leaves and stems are great for liver damage. Do not use the flowers.

Peppermint stimulates the liver.

Selenium is needed in cases of liver cirrhosis.

For a liver/pancreas stimulant, take ½ teaspoon nutmeg in 1 cup hot water.

Apricots detoxify the liver and pancreas.

Butternut is a liver food.

Stewed tomatoes are good for the liver.

– Lung –

*see also Asthma, Bronchial Trouble, Bronchitis, Cough, Emphysema, Respiratory
Fenugreek is useful for lung congestion.

Cabbage is anti-inflammatory and antibacterial, and is helpful in lung problems.

Thyme tea helps to relieve shortness of breath.

Cardamom also has a soothing effect on all membranes and the lungs.

For Pneumonia:
Hold right hand on forehead, left on back of head. Hold for fifteen minutes. ⤵

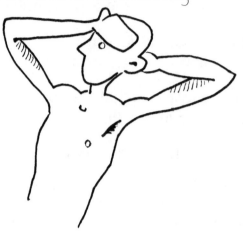

– **Lyme Disease** –

Make sure to see your physician for this disease. In addition, add Spirokete, and 2-34 Staph.

Lyme is a disease that is transmitted by ticks. Three to 32 days after being bitten by an infected tick, a skin lesion will appear. The lesion feels hot to the touch. Oftentimes there are attacks of arthritis, fatigue, chills, fever, stiff neck, sore muscles, nausea, and vomiting. ⤵

– **Lymph Ailments** –

Lettuce is great for swollen lymph glands.

Basil is also helpful to relieve swollen glands.

Barley is a calcium supplier and lymph cleanser, as well as a colon aid.

Cucumber juice, 4 to 5 cups a day, will purify the lymphatic system.

Two capsules twice a day of Echinacea will help a diseased lymph gland.

For enlarged lymph glands, take poke root tea.

Two cups a day of burdock root tea will help with lymphatic trouble.

Red beets will help people with lymph problems.

Bananas are loaded with potassium. We need potassium to keep the lymph system fit. ≋

~ Memory ~

*see also Brain, Forgetfulness

Almonds are excellent for the brain, 6 to 10 a day.

Almond oil improves the memory. Take 1 teaspoon a day.

Sage is a wonderful remedy for the memory. Use fresh sage in everything.

Four cloves in any tea mixture a day will heighten your memory.

Take three prunes a day to improve your memory.

Two mustard seeds a day will also help with your memory.

Ginkgo Biloba. ≋

~ **Menopause** ~

*see also Female Trouble
Cinnamon is very useful for menopausal difficulties and scanty menses.

Yams are beneficial to menopausal women. ⤳

~ **Menstrual** ~

*see also Female Trouble, PMS
Hot ginger tea helps to stimulate delayed menstrual periods and relieve menstrual cramps.

Okra has been found to be useful in cases of heavy menstrual bleeding.

Oregano is useful for menstrual pains.

The oil extracted from the seeds of borage is available in capsules and is used for menstrual problems.

Lemon balm has been used to relieve menstrual pain. ⤳

~ **Mercury in Tissues** ~

Selenium containing colloidal minerals is effective in removing mercury from the tissues.

Emu-mu counteracts mercury in the nervous system. ⤳

~ **Metallic Poison** ~

Green beans and zucchini eaten exclusively for three days will get rid of metallic poison.

Squash and strawberries remove arsenic poison, as well as other metallic poisons.

Wheat sprouts will improve detoxification of tissue and protect against heavy metal damage in the body.

Other helpful hints for metallic poisonings are as follows: Pumpkin seeds, rhubarb root, cayenne pepper, dulse, peppermint, vitamin C, Mexican raw sugar (1 tsp. several times a day), and Metaline™.

The following recipe removes lead from your tissue:

> 1 gallon cranberry juice
> 2 tbsp. whole cloves
> 2 tsp. ground cinnamon
> 1 tsp. cream of tartar

Directions: Boil the cloves in 1 quart cranberry juice for 20 minutes. Strain and add two tsp. ground cinnamon. Stir and add it to the rest of the cranberry juice. Now add 1 tsp. cream of tartar. Stir. Drink 5 ounces 3 times daily. For children, 3 ounces 3 times daily for 12–15 days. Then do it once a week.

~ **Migraines** ~

*see also Headaches

Magnesium is great for migraines.

Dioxin is a broad-leaf herbicide first widely used in Vietnam. It was one of the ingredients in a product called Agent Orange. It is now commonly used in the United States as a lawn and garden spray and for many commercial uses including the paper manufacturing process. Spraying our lawns causes exposure through both breathing the vapors and playing on the lawn, allows it to be absorbed through the skin, most commonly through the soles of the feet. We breathe it daily in the smog and pollution around industrial cities. It is also commonly found in corn and is often a factor in people who have corn allergies, causing migraine headaches. Dioxin settles in the brain, the digestive system, and sometimes the kidneys. Dioxin by itself is very toxic, but it is usually the cause or the catalyst of many other problems. Dioxin in the body attracts viruses, including Epstein Barr, parasites such as threadworm, whipworm, etc., and many other diseases and syndromes.

I know of only one antidote, and that is Homeopathic Dioxin.

~ **Milk Intolerance** ~

Parsnips are great for milk intolerance.

~ Miscarriage ~

Rosemary can be helpful to prevent miscarriage.

Apple tree bark tea will check miscarriages.

~ Mononucleosis ~

Red raspberry leaf tea can help with mono-nucleosis.

Leaf lettuce water/tea is also helpful for mono.

Use raw tomato poultices to the neck for swelling induced by mononucleosis.

~ Morning Sickness ~

*see also Pregnancy

Peach tree leaves are great for morning sick-ness.

~ Mouth ~

*see also Gum Problems, Teeth

When the tongue adheres to the roof of the mouth, take nutmeg.

Savory makes an excellent antiseptic mouth-wash and gargle.

Myrrh seems to help mouth conditions such as gum infections, gingivitis, sore throats, and mouth ulcers.

For canker sores, wrap finely grated carrot with cloth and lay against canker sore. Change every 2 hours.

Sage can also be used as a mouthwash and is helpful with sore throats, gum disease, and mouth ulcers.

For mouth burning, drink and hold poppy seed tea in mouth several times a day.

For a dry mouth, chew a small piece of calamus root.

For mouth odor, chew juniper berries or gargle with rosemary tea.

For mouth ulcers, chew sage or willow leaves, or hold blackberry leaf tea in mouth.

When the corners of the mouth are cracked, take zinc.

For involuntary dribbling of saliva, please give selenium.

Gum Infection (Gingivitis):
Take 2 ounces mulberry twigs and cut them in little pieces. Boil the pieces in 1 quart of white grape juice for 30 minutes. Let it cool and then take 1 tablespoon every 2 hours. Swish it in your mouth before you swallow it. One quart will do.

Tongue Problems:
For sores on the tongue, hold raspberry leaf tea in mouth several times a day.

For a burning tongue, boil and hold a teaspoon of malva in mouth.

‒ **Mucous Conditions** ‒

Oranges are great mucous cleansers for stomach, ears, head, and sinuses, but only if taken as follows: Drink 1 glass fresh orange juice and the same amount of distilled water, but do not mix. Drink the orange juice, then follow with the water. Do this as often as wanted, 10 times a day more or less. No other food should be taken. Do this for 2 days in a row 2–3 times a year.

Fenugreek is one of the oldest medicinal plants and is a versatile spice. The Egyptians valued fenugreek for eating, healing, and embalming. It is useful for mucous conditions.

‒ **Multiple Sclerosis** ‒

Multiple sclerosis happens when the nerve casings, known as myelin sheaths, lose their protective outer fatty layer that insulates the nerves themselves and increases the speed of electrical transmissions. In MS, some parts of these sheaths are destroyed and replaced by scar tissue. This process, called sclerosis, occurs at various sites throughout the central nervous system. Some of the most common symptoms include extreme fatigue, muscle spasms, blurred and double vision, numbness in the extremities, loss of coordination, mental confusion, and paralysis.

To help, make a tea of sunflower seeds and fenugreek seeds. Drink one cup, three times daily.

Another remedy is to make a smoothie with corn, grated carrots, liquid garlic, chives, milk, dry mustard, paprika, flaxseed oil, and primrose oil. Place it all in a blender, and add salt or pepper to taste.

Emu-mu drops will help rebuild the central nervous system.

– Muscles –

Beef is a muscle food.

Beans and corn are muscle builders. Try beans and cornbread.

Try buckwheat for strong muscles.

Rye is also a muscle builder.

Red beans are a muscle builder. Served with corn, it is a complete protein.

Use magnesium for aches in the shoulder muscle.

Use vitamin B_1, B_2, E, and calcium lactate for cramps in the muscles.

Lathyrus-Chick Pea Homeopathic will help with very tense calves.

Two cups a day of shepherd's purse tea will help with deterioration of the muscles.

Vitamin E is needed for good muscle function.

Magnesium is needed for jerks in the muscles.

Vitamins E, B, and calcium lactate are great for pain in the muscles.

For spasms in the muscles, try calcium lactate, especially when the spasms are at night.

For daytime spasms, try magnesium.

Skullcap will help with twitching of the muscles.

Eat almonds for weakness in muscles, especially after an illness.

Soak 1 teaspoon chia seed in 4 ounces juice for 2–3 hours, and drink 3–4 times a day for muscle strength.

Use buckwheat in your foods to help strengthen muscles.

For muscle weakness, take a handful of apple peelings, boil in one quart water for 20 minutes, strain, and drink 6 ounces daily.

Use comfrey compresses for muscle injuries, especially in the tendons and tissues.

Also try arnica tincture compresses, or take arnica by mouth for muscle injuries.

Daisy tea is great for muscle injuries. Drink 2–3 cups a day.

Gentian tea is a treatment for general muscle weakness. Drink ½ cup a day.

Wormwood with lady's mantle tea is also great for muscle weakness.

For muscle weakness in children, try barley malt.

Children can also benefit from juniper berry branches. Boil for 45 minutes, strain, then add the tea to bath water. Soak for 20 minutes.

For muscle weakness in senior citizens, try 2 cups of yarrow tea a day.

Biotin is also beneficial for muscle pain and weakness.

Marjoram can relieve muscle spasms.

Baptisia and Arsenicum Homeopathic will help with soreness in muscles.

~ Nausea ~

*see also Travel Sickness, Vomiting
Peppermint does an excellent job in reducing nausea.

Ginger can also help with nausea.

Cinnamon is good to relieve nausea and vomiting.

The flowers and oil of cloves are used to remove nausea and vomiting.

Nutmeg aids nausea.

Lemon balm is also used for nausea.

~ Nerves ~

Blanched almonds with grapes assist nerves

Eat tender celery to help depleted nerves.

Pineapple juice mixed with prune juice rebuilds exhausted nerves. Drink 6 ounces 3 times a day.

Try 2 egg yolks mixed with 4 ounces grape juice once or twice daily for a great nerve food.

Another great nerve food is applewhey. Take 1 pint apple juice and mix with 1 pint water and 1 pint milk. Heat slowly, but do not boil. When it curdles, strain through a fine cloth. Discard curds. Sweeten mixture with honey, and take 2 tablespoons 5 times a day.

Myrtle is a nerve sedative.

~ Nervous Conditions ~

*see also Anxiety

Sesame seeds can help to prevent nervous breakdowns.

Oat water added to fruit juice is a great nerve tonic.

Barley water added to fruit juice is also a great nerve tonic.

For nervous complaints, try 2 cups of motherwort tea a day.

Valerian root taken ½ cup twice a day will also help with nervous complaints.

For nervous exhaustion, try silicon herbs.

Rue tea is great for a nervous heart, but do not take during pregnancy.

Catnip is great for nervous tension.

Mint will also help with nervous tension. Drink 1 cup as needed.

Bugleweed tea is beneficial for nervousness.

Caraway is very much like anise and when mixed with anise is twice as good. It is used for nervous conditions.

Marjoram has been used for nervous disorders.

Sage tea helps the body and nervous system relax.

Ginseng will help an involuntary nervous system.

Horsetail tea will also help an involuntary nervous system.

For nervousness, try mixing hops, St. John's wort, and rosemary. Mix, make a tea, and drink 2 cups a day.

Many nerve diseases have kidney trouble.

~ Neuralgia ~

Vitamin B-complex is needed to aid neuralgia.

Boil the crushed fruit of allspice, and apply on a cloth to aid neuralgia.

~ Neuritis ~

Combine avocado with agar-agar (dry), lime juice, and raw rolled oats. Drink plenty of distilled water between meals. ⤚

~ Nightmares ~

A sprig of rosemary under the pillow has been known to alleviate children's nightmares. ⤚

~ Numbness ~

Numbness in the lower lip is remedied by a sprinkle of anise or anise tea. ⤚

~ Obesity ~

*see also Overweight

Celery is a low-calorie food that can aid in losing weight.

Drink the tea of celery seed to help with obesity.

The entire plant or only the seeds of fennel will help with obesity.

Fennel is one of the oldest cultivated plants and was highly valued by the Romans. The warriors used it to maintain good health, and the women ate it to prevent obesity. ⤚

~ Overweight ~

*see also Obesity

Simmer one teaspoon fennelseed in 8 ounces water for 10 minutes. Drink 3 to 4 cups a day for overweight problems.

Use 1 teaspoon gelatin with each meal. Some overweight people need glycine, which happens to be in gelatin.

~ Pain ~

Epsom salt can help to relieve pain in hands and feet. Put about 1 tablespoon of Epsom salt in warm water and soak for about 20 minutes.

Aconite (Aconitum napellus), comfrey (Symphytum officinale), chicory (Cichorium intybus), and English mandrake (Tamus communis) will help with pain.

Try eating a piece of grapefruit if you have pain in the temporal region.

Cabbage is good for aches and pains.

Cinnamon can help such pains as lower back, abdominal, and heart pain.

Alfalfa contains many trace minerals and, when used as a tea, releases pain in the head and limbs.

Horseradish is used as a pain reliever for neck and back pain when taken internally.

Coriander as an oil can be rubbed on for painful and rheumatic joints. It is cooling, soothing, and calming to the body.

Yams are great for any kind of pain.

For pain in the Achilles tendon, try Homeopathic St. John's Wort.

For pain in ankles and feet, drink 2 cups or soak feet in poke root tea.

For ankle joint pain try Homeopathic Tiger Lily.

Comfrey root tincture applied to the painful area will also help.

For breathing pain, try taking more iron.

For burning pain, use vitamin B_{12} and folic acid.

For cramp-like pain in feet and soles, try mullein leaf tea or cabbage compresses.

For pain deep in the head, try buckwheat in your food.

For facial pain, use vitamin B_{12} and folic acid.

For acute finger pain, use St. John's wort.

For pain from hip to feet, use cayenne pepper in socks.

For radiating head pain, drink 1 cup of black tea.

For head pain with nausea, try Homeopathic Iris-Blue Flag.

For nerve pain in head, try lady's slipper tea, lavender tea, or lavender oil applied to temples.

For headaches, try 1 cup of guarana tea.

Lavender oil is great for any local pain when applied.

Echinacea tea or in capsules is great for pectoral muscle pain.

Horsetail tea or in capsules is great for cramp-like rheumatic pain.

Take yucca tablets for pain in the right side of liver area.

For shifting pain, use poke root tea or yams.

For spinal pain, use pink root as a tea, ½ cup twice daily.

For pain in the shoulder, try iron, copper, vitamin B_1, or folic acid.

For amputated stump pain, use vitamin B_1 and vitamin B_{12}.

For pain in the toes, use St. John's wort.

For wandering nature pain use echinacea.

Strawberries contain organic salicylates. These are the active ingredient in aspirin.

Pour three pounds Epsom salt into bath, and soak for ½ hour until pain recedes.

When salt is heated in a frying pan and prepared in a cloth sack, and put on painful area, it is very helpful. Cover this with hot water bottle.

~ **Pancreas Problems** ~

Blueberries and bananas are great for pancreatitis.

Green beans are good for the malfunctions of the pancreas.

½ teaspoon of nutmeg is great for the pancreas.

Stewed tomatoes will cleanse the pancreas when combined with lime.

Apricots are splendid for detoxifying the liver and the pancreas.

Selenium is needed in the cases of pancreatic atrophy.

Cucumber contains a hormone needed by the pancreas for insulin production.

For a liver-pancreas stimulant, take ½ tsp. nutmeg in 1 cup hot water. This causes the pancreas to release juices and will build the liver.

Use 1 drop of iodine in 1 glass of water for pancreas trouble which can be detected by the sense of oppression in the stomach region. The sensation is as if there were a morsel stuck in the throat.

To strengthen the pancreas, boil green beans in plenty of water. Drink one cup of bean water a day, and eat one cup of green beans a day.

Pancreatic flukes are serious. Take Homeopathic Pancreatic Flukes to help.

~ **Parasites** ~

Garlic is anti-parasitic and helps the body rid itself of worms and other parasites. Take 3 cloves of garlic, boil in 1 cup of milk, for 5 minutes. Let it cool enough to drink and strain, drink this every night for 10 nights in a row.

To keep parasites out of your body, take 2 tsps. of apple cider vinegar every day in 6 to 7 ounces water.

To treat tapeworm, take 5 parts juniper berries and 5 parts white oil for one day.

Pomegranate is also helpful to expel tapeworms from the body.

Calcanea will also help with worms.

Thyme has been used to treat parasites such as roundworms, tapeworms, threadworms, and hookworms.

Lima bean pods and peach tree leaves will help to alleviate microscopic parasites.

For ringworm, rub banana peel on the area.

Cloves will also help to expel worms.

Pumpkin is a de-wormer as well as pancreas food.

Pumpkin seeds are used to rid the body of parasites.

~ Parkinson's Disease ~

This condition is characterized by the inability to control movements, as in hands, arms, and speech. Your physician will treat this with L-Dopa. L-Dopa helps the nervous system. However, Parkinson's disease has proven to be a disease of the central nervous system.

Emu-mu (an oil made from the emu bird and other special oils) removes the blockage from the central nervous system in a short time.

This Emu-mu oil can be used for people who suffer from any kind of shaking disease, or shaking from old age. It will help clear the central nervous system and help the shaking stop.

~ Piles ~

*see also Hemorrhoids

Dates and milk instead of breakfast will help with piles.

Take vitamin B$_6$.

~ Pinkeye ~

*see also Eye Problems

Soak a clean washcloth in warm water and apply to the eyes as a compress for a few minutes, several times a day. Be sure to wash anything that comes in contact with your eyes thoroughly and often. If pinkeye, or conjunctivitis, doesn't clear up in a few days, you should see your doctor.

~ Pituitary Problems ~

Watercress will help with pituitary problems. Alternate one bunch of watercress a day, next day six ounces pineapple juice two times a day.

Wild cherry bark tincture, seven drops twice daily.

~ PMS ~

*see also Female Trouble, Menstrual
Calcium and magnesium are great for PMS sufferers.

Also try black cohosh for PMS.

Feed your adrenal glands.

~ Poison Oak ~

Homeopathic Anacardium is an antidote for poison oak.

Rub cream of tartar over it.

~ Pregnancy ~

*see also Morning Sickness
Coconut water should be drunk by pregnant women on an empty stomach, in the morning. This will bring clear urine and will greatly nourish the fetus.

Peaches are good during pregnancy.

Ginger will help with sickness during pregnancy.

~ **Prostate** ~

Foon Goos #2 and Men's Special™ will help with all prostate problems.

Zinc will also help with the prostate.

Bee pollen can help with the prostate.

Saw palmetto tincture is also believed to help with the prostate.

Myrrh is thought to cleanse the prostate system and balance hypothyroid problems.

Coconut will help to nourish the prostate gland and the testicles and removes heat or burning sensation from these organs.

Pumpkin seeds can bring relief to prostate trouble.

~ **Psoriasis** ~

Cool baths with apple cider vinegar added to the water brings relief.

~ **Pus Diseases** ~

Homeopathic Hypericum will help with pus.

Vinegar is good in all pus diseases. Take one quart water, 2 tablespoons vinegar, heat, and inhale vapor for 10 minutes 3–4 times a day for pus formations of lungs, sinuses, and throat.

~ **Radiation** ~

*see also Fallout

Radioactive chemical released from the nuclear power and weapons industry, combined with other industrial pollution, cause a problem known as fallout. Each day, down through the atmosphere, these pollutants flow, causing a wide variety of symptoms including:

>   anxiety
>   hysteria
>   insatiable hunger
>   extreme nervousness
>   feeling of unreality
>   dizziness and vertigo
>   rheumatic pains
>   hearing problems
>   complete exhaustion
>   extreme tiredness
>   pendulous mood swings
>   hot and cold flashes
>   loss of will power
>   gastric distress
>   extreme headache
>   aches in the joints
>   memory loss
>   sore throat

This damage is widespread. Fallout affects all of us. It lingers in the vegetables, the plants, on the animals, etc. When it rains or snows, we get extra doses of it. Here are a few of the methods used to counteract fallout:

1) 1 tsp. baking soda, 1 tsp. sea salt, ½ tsp. cream of tartar, one quart of water. Mix and drink 8 ounces every two hours.
2) Homeopathic "R.A. Fallout."
3) According to Dr. Carl C. Pfeifer, to help overcome pollution, he recommends this combination of nutrients taken together: Lysine, Cystine, Methionine.
4) After the nuclear accident in Russia, vitamin B_{15} was given to the population to counteract the fallout, and they had good results with it.
5) The herb combination of willow leaves, milksugar, thyme, and cinnamon. The trade name is "Pol-X." See your health food store.
6) Also, three herbs have been very helpful: ginseng, valerian root, and passa flora (passion flower).

It is also known that the vitamins A, B-complex, and C are helpful to overcome the effects of fallout and radiation.

~ Respiratory ~

*see also Asthma, Bronchial Trouble, Bronchitis, Cough, Emphysema, Lung

Honey can be beneficial for respiratory problems and can relieve cough and sore throats. For fever, drink hot lemon juice with honey.

Celery has been found to be beneficial for respiratory ailments. Eating fresh stalks of celery after childbirth can help stimulate milk production. Celery juice is very helpful for joint inflammation, rheumatoid arthritis, and nervous exhaustion.

Marjoram can be calming to the respiratory system.

Violet leaves and chickweed for respiratory problems may also be helpful.

~ Restless Leg Syndrome ~

This condition relates to folic acid deficiency. If possible, give vitamin E-rich foods. Also lack of tryptophan leads to restless leg syndrome. Since this restlessness makes insomnia, it is good to know that people can sleep after a few days on amino acids.

~ Rheumatism ~

Marjoram tea or oil put into bath water can relieve rheumatism and tension. Put a drop of marjoram oil on the pillow to induce sleep. Its aromatic influences are said to be peaceful and to help induce sleep.

Rosemary stimulates circulation and eases pain by increasing the flow of blood where applied. It is used for aching joints and rheumatism.

Oregano has been used for irritability, exhaustion, and as a sedative. It is thought to prevent seasickness. It can be applied externally for swelling, rheumatism, and a stiff neck.

The oil extracted from the seeds of borage is available in capsules and is used for rheumatic disorders.

Combine avocado with agar-agar (dry), lime juice and raw rolled oats. Drink plenty of distilled water between meals.

Celery increases appetite, is good in curing mucus and therefore is used in rheumatic pain.

Boil the crushed fruit of allspice and apply on a cloth to aid rheumatism and neuralgia.

Basil eases the pain in rheumatism. Drink it as a tea and/or sprinkle it on an oiled cloth, and apply to aching parts.

Raw potatoes carried in your pocket until they are shriveled up and stink from the poison can help with rheumatism. Carry the raw potato in your pocket for several days, then repeat.

Sawdust has natural D.M.S.O. Take pine sawdust, boil it in water for ten minutes, and place hands or feet into warm mush. When in spine, strain mush and place in sack.

~ Scabies ~

Thyme tea has been used as a skin antiseptic for scabies.

~ Scars ~

Homeopathics Drosera Silica and Graphite are used for scars.

Vitamin E taken externally and applied to the scar may also be helpful.

Apply pure cocoabutter to the scar to help reduce it.

~ Sciatica ~

Elderberry juice is terrific for sciatica and facial twitching.

Used as a poultice of hot milk and crushed seeds, fenugreek relieves sciatica.

~ Scurvy ~

Scurvy/bleeding gums, is caused by a vitamin C deficiency. Scurvy may also occur concurrently with gingivitis.

Treatment of scurvy should include vitamin C to bowel tolerance, increase green leafy vegetables and fruit intake, and herbs including dog rose, also known as Rosa canina.

~ Shingles ~

*see also Skin

If every scratch becomes a sore, peppermint tea is helpful. It can be used as an eyewash for inflammations and as a wash for skin ailments like itching, burns, ringworm, and bug bites.

Peppermint can be used for shingles, as well as infected or painful nerves. For vaginal itching, use a very mild tea of peppermint as a douche to bring relief.

Homeopathic Arsenicum Metallicum, also known as metallic arsenic, can also be used for shingles.

One and one half quarts of celery juice daily can help with shingles.

Make a paste of Epsom salts by adding water to make the right consistency, then apply frequently to the affected parts until relief is met.

Also Homeopathic Ranunculus will help.

~ Shock ~

Eating oranges helps calm the nerves and is useful for shock.

Hypericum or St. John's wort will also help with shock.

~ Sinus Problems ~

Horseradish plant is widely used in the southern part of Germany. It is given when frontal bones hurt, for sinus trouble, and for salivary gland difficulties. In this region, people gargle with horseradish broth if they have throat problems, hoarseness, or hearing problems.

For sinus problems or an infection in the sinuses, take 1 tsp. of honey, sprinkle with freshly ground black pepper, and eat.

Horseradish, onion, turnips, mustard, and radishes also help with sinus problems.

Take a piece of fresh horseradish, or open a jar of horseradish relish, and take a little piece several times a day.

Garlic is nature's antibiotic, and if added to your diet, it will make mucus less sticky and will help fight the infection.

~ Skin ~

*see also Acne, Dermatitis, Eczema, Shingles
Cucumbers are a delightful vegetable with many medicinal uses. Cucumbers are very good for the skin, especially the complexion. Either eaten or used topically, they cool and heal the skin.

One third teaspoon of freshly ground nutmeg, one teaspoon of honey, and four or five ounces hot water taken three mornings in a row, then a three-day break, then repeated nine times, can help with boils and pimples of the skin.

For facial pimples, make a mask of Epsom salts and water and pat on the afflicted area with cotton before going to bed. Do this every night until pimples are gone.

Thuja, Staph, or Arsenicum Homeopathics are great for skin problems.

Coconut oil is very good for massage on the scalp. It can be massaged all over the body in summer. It agrees with fire constitution. Oil is applied with success on skin troubles like itching, eczema, dermatitis, etc. The oil is used for frying and cooking purposes in South India.

Used fresh on the skin, garlic has been known to heal acne and other skin problems. Rubbing raw garlic on warts and corns is said to heal them. It promotes sweating and acts like an antihistamine. Rubbing garlic directly on an insect sting relieves pain as well.

Myrrh has been found by the Arabic people to help skin conditions such as athlete's foot, eczema, cracked skin, ringworm, and wrinkles. It was also used for asthma, coughs, and bronchitis.

Make a salve of soybean lecithin for red, itchy, scaly skin, as in psoriasis, and also take 2 tablespoons by mouth.

Parsley can be chewed raw to freshen the breath and promote healthy skin. Eating parsley after garlic or onion will help deodorize the breath and the body.

For the disease called shingles, use common Epsom salts, making a paste of it by adding water to the right consistency, then apply frequently to the affected parts until relief is achieved. This happens in a very short time.

Walnut leaves are also used for acne on the face.

Dandelion is also used for acne.

Nettle and strawberry leaves, used singly or together as a tea, can help with acne.

Strawberry leaf tea is used for eczema.

Club moss behind the ear is also great for eczema.

Pansy tea (Violet triealas) can be used for eczema in childhood.

Evening primrose oil can be used for eczema, eruptions, and blisters. Use on joints and fingers.

For a splinter, rub onion on the area. Also, use onion poultice on a boil to bring it to a head.

For skin blemishes, make a paste of spirits of camphor in soda bicarb. Pat on area and leave on overnight. Use for one week.

Cucumber is a very good diuretic. Cucumber contains a hormone needed by the pancreas to produce insulin. It is specific for skin troubles.

To remove a splinter with no pain, freeze the area with an ice cube first.

For extremely chapped hands and skin, mix three drops of lemon oil and three drops glycerin, and apply to the irritated area for fast relief.~

~ Sleep Apnea ~

*see also Sleeping Disorders
Vitamin B_1 is good for sleep apnea.~

~ Sleeping Disorders ~

*see also Sleep Apnea and Insomnia
Simmer dill seeds in olive oil and rub this oil on the forehead for better sleeping.

Nutmeg tea inspires sleep and is thought to overcome frigidity, impotence, and nervous fatigue. Use this spice sparingly because large doses can be poisonous and can cause a miscarriage.

Alfalfa is also used to induce sleep.~

~ Slow Learning Children ~

Slow learning children benefit from alfalfa with dill.~

~ Smoking Habit ~

The herb calamus root has been found to rebuild the lung from smoking damage. Use the following recipe:

One quart apple juice
One rounded teaspoon calamus root
Boil both together for 15 minutes, strain, and
drink six ounces of it, three times daily.

Parsley, carrots, and celery protect against cer-
tain carcinogens found in tobacco smoke and
help regulate prostaglandin production. The active food component in these foods are called
"polyacetylenes."

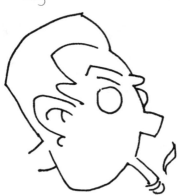

– Sores –

Put honey on sores, and they will heal quickly.
It is antiseptic and antibacterial. During war
shortages, honey was often used with oil or lard
as a dressing for small wounds or ulcers. It was
so used in Shanghai during World War II.

– Sore Throat –

In ancient Egypt, women burned myrrh to
get rid of fleas in their homes. It has a particu-

larly unpleasant taste, but has been found to be excellent for sore throats and mouth ulcers. (Use as a gargle.)

Peppermint is also used to soothe sore throats and is antibacterial. For sinus problems, drink lots of peppermint tea and apply a large warm peppermint pack to the sinus area for immediate relief.

To relieve a sore throat, soak a cotton cloth in marjoram tea and wrap it around the throat. Wrap another, larger cloth over it, making it as airtight as possible, and leave on several hours or overnight.

Homeopathic St. Ignatius Bean can be helpful for a lump in the throat also known as *Globus hystericus.*

Blue malva is also used for lumps in the throat.

A tea made with hot water and licorice root is very soothing to a sore throat.

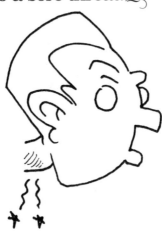

– **Spleen** –

Eggplant is food for the spleen. Eat two to three small pieces of cooked eggplant before breakfast on an empty stomach to reduce an enlarged spleen, and increase red blood corpuscles and hemoglobin. Eggplant is also very good for anemia.

Okra is food for the spleen.

Yams have been used for ailments of the kidneys, lung, and stomach, as well as for urinary infections and asthma, spleen, and stomach.

Beets are also food for the spleen.

For an enlarged spleen, take homeopathic Chionoutus-Fringe Tree.

Not only is the red beet noted for its rich mineral content, but it is betaine, a red pigment that increases oxidation within body cells. Betaine acts as a methyl donor much in the same way that Pangamic Acid does. The structure of betaine is similar to lecithin and is found in muscle tissue and is a building block for important factors related to the health of the liver, kidneys, spleen, and pancreas.

Have a chiropractor release the tension in the tailbone and lumbar region.

Do not massage!

~ Sprue ~

*see Celiac Disease

~ Staph Infection ~

Savory is antibacterial, antifungal, and anti-viral and has been used to treat staph infection.

Oxoquiniline from the quinine tree can also be helpful for staph infections.

Homeopathic Staph is the only one *I* depend on.

~ Stiff Neck ~

For a stiff neck, you need a liver remedy, which is Homeopathic Cheladonium or Livah, an herb formula.

Also for a stiff neck, check always for female trouble.

~ Stomach Ailments ~

Ginger tea is great for stomach ailments. Here is the recipe:

Use 1 to 2 teaspoons of granulated Jamaican ginger to 2 cups of boiling water. Pour the hot water over the ginger. Cover the container and allow the tea to steep until sufficiently cool to drink. Drink ½ to 1 cup at a time. Ginger tea may be flavored with a few cloves or a dash of nutmeg.

Hot compresses of ginger tea on the stomach will relieve cramping. It is helpful for stomach flu, both as a tea to drink and as a compress on the stomach.

Ginger tea is also indicated for confusion, debility, and cramps in soles of feet or palms of hands. When joints feel weak or there is a heavy feeling in the stomach, ginger tea will bring relief. It relieves hoarseness and asthma without anxiety. When there is intestinal catarrh, painful and hot hemorrhoids, or a painful anus, ginger tea will help.

Rosemary is for weak stomachs.

Pumpkin is high in beta carotene and is, therefore, an excellent food. It calms an upset stomach.

For ulceration of the stomach, okra and apples are used.

Green and dried peas are a good source of protein and good for weak stomachs.

Pineapple is an enzyme supplier good for stomachs.

Red beets are good for stomach ailments.

One tablespoon whey, three times daily, will feed the stomach glands and they will work better for you.

Cardamom has a soothing effect on all membranes, including the stomach and lungs. ∽

– **Stone and Gout** –

*see also Gout

A good recipe for stone and gout is as follows:

1 quart apple cider
1 teaspoon hydrangea root

Let these stand for twelve hours, bring to a boil, simmer. Take ½ cup three times daily.

Here is another marvelous recipe to lubricate joints and make joints supple. A young girl, a flower child, gave it to me. I wish I could show to everyone the lovely drawing she put under the recipe.

1 teaspoon turmeric
2 teaspoons almond oil
2 tablespoons soy milk powder
1 cup water
salt and honey to taste

Heat this and serve as a lovely hot drink. ∽

– **Strep** –

Cucumbers are good for strep.

For a strep infection, take Homeopathic Ailanthus Glandulosa (Chinese sumach). ∽

– **Stress** –

Stress comes from an unnatural and negative environment. Denatured food, widespread poisons such as dioxin (Agent Orange), m.s.g., etc., produce physical stress within the body, while cement, metal, and asphalt produce an external physical stress, which disturbs our work and family life. We need a release from this negativity.

Borage has also been thought to be helpful when taken as a tincture for stress.

Lemon balm helps indigestion especially during worry or anxiety.

Take nutritional supplements, including extra magnesium orotate, B_{15}, lecithin, vitamin E, zinc, manganese, selenium, garlic, and cod-liver oil at bedtime (also good for heart disease).

– Sugar Craving –

To help ease the craving for sugar, rub the elbows in a clockwise motion:

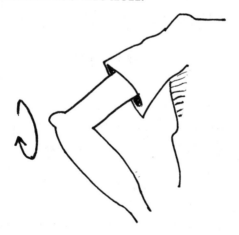

Clean pancreas from worms (flukes).

– **Suicidal Tendency** –

Make two cups or more black tea and add sugar or honey for suicidal tendencies.

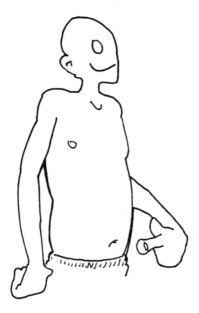

If you are seriously depressed, just press your belly button.

– **Sunburn** –

Aloe vera is great for sunburns.

Cornstarch mixed with water to make a paste and applied directly to the sunburn will help ease the pain.

Boil lettuce leaves, strain, and let the liquid cool several hours in the refrigerator. Apply gently to the sunburned areas.

Yogurt or cooled tea bags applied to a sunburn will help decrease the swelling of a sunburn. ⌒

~ Swelling ~

A slice of tomato on swelling reduces it quickly.

Lettuce water can be applied externally over swollen parts of the body such as ankles, abdomen, and liver.

For swollen glands, you can make a compress with baked banana in the skin, mashed with a little fresh cream or olive oil.

Cabbage is terrific for poultices over swollen knees or elbows. Grate two cups of cabbage very fine. Wrap in a cloth and apply overnight to swollen knees or ankles. Do this several days in a row for best results.

Simmer one handful of potato peelings in two cups water for 15 minutes. Strain and take two tablespoons of this in a glass of water for fourteen days. After several days, your legs and ankles should be at a more normal size. Do this 3 times daily.

Boil adzuki beans in plenty of water. Eat them as a soup, or drink the fluid two times daily for swelling. ⌒

~ Teeth ~

*see also Gum Problems, Mouth, Toothache
Chewing on an oregano leaf provides temporary relief for a toothache.

Used as a mouthwash, fennel is thought to help loose teeth, gum disorders, laryngitis, and sore throats. Its aromatic influences increase longevity, courage, and purification.

Simmer 1 teaspoon fennel seeds in 1 cup of water for 10 minutes. Drink 3 to 4 cups daily to balance obese conditions. Additionally, fennel seeds can be added to salads to ease this condition. This tea is also excellent in conditions of colds and flu.

Citrus fruits, licorice root extract, soy products, and curcumin prevent dental decay. The active food component is Triterpenoids.

Soak a piece of cotton in the oil of cloves and place in the dental cavity to subside the pain.

Nutmeg oil can be applied to aching teeth with a cotton swab until dental treatment is available.

Eat aged cheese, such as cheddar, before meals to stop the formation of plaque before it starts.

– Tissue –

Cabbage is used as a tissue builder which contains vitamin U.

Leeks, a pancreas food, builds tissue and is brain food.

Lemon (the white) is a bioflavonoid and strengthens tissue.

Garlic helps reduce carbohydrate residue in tissue and glands.

A universal acceptance by all tissues is rice, which is overrated at the present time.

For tissue swelling, juniper berries help reduce tissue swelling.

~ Tonsils ~

Don't eat bananas if you have a cold or cough, as they will add to the problems. You can make a compress for swollen tonsils with banana baked in the skin, mashed with a little fresh cream or olive oil.

Savory tea can be used as an antiseptic mouthwash and gargle for tonsils.

~ Toothache ~

*see also Teeth

Cayenne can be rubbed on a toothache and used for swelling and inflammation. When cayenne tincture is rubbed on an arthritic joint and wrapped with flannel cloth overnight, the pain is usually gone by morning.

Cloves help to relieve toothaches. Insert a little oil of cloves into the cavity, or roll a bruised clove around in the mouth. To make oil of cloves, take a handful of cloves, bruise them, pack them into a jar, and cover with olive oil until the jar is full.

Strain the oil after one week. Save the oil, and add fresh cloves. This can be repeated as often as necessary until the oil is saturated with cloves.

For loose teeth, drink 3 cups of parsley tea a day.

Epsom salts are a good cleanser. Pour 3 lbs. Epsom salts into your bathtub. Add hot water as you like it and soak for ½ hour. All pains will be gone. A weak solution for weak gums and painful teeth, just hold the warm solution in your mouth.

Cabbage is also good for teeth.

– **Tranquilizer** –

The word "dill" comes from the Saxon word "to lull," because it has many tranquilizing effects. Dill is very useful for its high natural mineral salt content.

– **Travel Sickness** –

*see also Nausea, Vomiting
Ginger is effective for travel sickness.

– **Triglycerides (elevated)** –

Elevated triglycerides can be a sign of diabetes or liver problems. Also, it is a high risk factor for cardiovascular disease and stroke.

To treat elevated triglyceride levels, do moderate exercise, avoid sugar, eat a high fiber diet, and eliminate red meat.

~ **Tumors** ~

Tomatoes, including tomato juice, contain lycopene, which is a substance known to reduce tumors.

Eggplant skin is very important in the treatment of tumors. Peel the eggplant ½ inch thick (leaving ½ inch of the meat). Boil, steam, or broil these peelings until soft. Season with kelp or dulse. This remedy relieves tumors and cellulite. Enjoy!

Recently it was found that turmeric contains a substance which significantly reduces the long-term recurrence of viruses. It also halts tumor and growth. Just use a small amount.

Asparagus can be used for fatty tumors and the like. It is also helpful in urinary secretions.

Turnips are used for deep-rooted tumors. Also for deep-rooted resentments.

Dr. Pearlstein from Israel recommends raw tomatoes applied to the head in case of tumors in the brain.

Eggplant enjoys a noteworthy position in vegetables. Known throughout the world, it is highly nutritious and a tonic. Eggplant has to be sliced and placed in slightly salted water for about 20 minutes or more. This will remove the bitterness.

General bad natured tumors can benefit from prickly pear.

Milkweed juice applied to the lips can help tumors on the lips.

Tea made from houseleek and cottonwood leaves can help bad-natured tumors of the breast.

Grapes are helpful with tumors.

Flax oil is beneficial for simple tumors.

– Ulcer –

Ginger is a blessing to an upset stomach. A pinch of ginger (about ¼ teaspoon) to about 6 ounces of hot water is sufficient to bring relief. Ginger has long been known for its soothing effect to the stomach and has frequently been added to other herbs to act as a buffer in the stomach.

Fenugreek is helpful in relieving ulcers and other inflamed conditions of the stomach and intestines. It relieves fever, diarrhea, and gas. It is used in the treatment of diabetes and gout and is an excellent tonic and rejuvenator.

Cooked carrots relieve stomach ulcers.

Calamus root tea is good for duodenal ulcers. The root should stand in water overnight. Warm it the next morning (do not boil). Drink ½ cup four to five times daily.

Red potatoes are also good for stomach and duodenal ulcers.

Peptic ulcers (gastric ulcer) are thought to be caused by stress, deficiency of vitamin U and/or dyspepsia. Symptoms of peptic ulcer include burning stomach pain, dyspepsia, and weight loss. "Coffee ground" stool indicates that the ulcer is bleeding and that the patient is in imminent danger of bleeding to death. (Go to a hospital IMMEDIATELY!)

Treatment of peptic ulcer should include alfalfa (Medicago sativa), which is thought to be the richest source of vitamin U at ten tablets t.i.d. with meals, cabbage juice (Brassica oleracea), flax (Linum usitatissimum), German chamomile (Matricaria chamomilla), and licorice (Glycyrrhiza glabra).

For ulceration of intestines, use potatoes, garlic, and golden seal.

For ulceration of the stomach, use okra, apples, and string beans.

Cabbage is helpful in hyperactivity and gastric ulcers.

Homeopathic Carbo Vegetabilis-Charcoal is also helpful.

Homeopathic Caruid Marians and St. Mary's thistle can also be used.

Citrus food, licorice root extract, and tritezsenoids are anti-ulcer agents.

Cabbage juice (freshly made) is used for stomach ulcers because of the vitamin U in cabbage.

Raw and cooked apples can be helpful for stomach ulcers.

Cooked okra, not heavily seasoned, can benefit stomach ulcers.

Juice one potato and add the same amount of warm water. Drink before each meal, three times daily for ulcers. Red potatoes are best.

– Urinary Tract –

To promote the free flow of urine, combine fennel seeds with caraway seed and juniper and drink the tea.

There are two varieties of coconut, one containing kernel or malai. They are sweet in nature. Therefore, they are more suitable to people having fire or pitta element. The other type, which hardly contains any kernel, is slightly salty in taste and is good for flushing the urinary system. It purifies the blood. In India, coconuts are available in plenty in the Malabar area near the seashore, and in this tropical country coconut plays a very important role.

Cherry juice is good when people urinate constantly. Some folks have to get up nights many times. A glass of cherry juice 3–4 times daily will help this trouble. Cherry juice stops constant urination.

For bleeding in the urine, combine 2 teaspoons each of comfrey root, dandelion root, and marshmallow root to one cup of water. Make a tea and drink.

Artichokes bring clear urine and are useful for albumin in the urine.

Celery increases appetite and is good in curing mucous conditions. Therefore it is used in urinary disorders.

Ginger also helps in urinary difficulties.

Juniper berries impart the smell of violets in the urine.

– Vaccinations –

For ill effects of vaccinations, use Homeopathic Thuja.

– Varicose Veins –

For varicose veins, use Homeopathic Arsenicum Metallicum

For varicose veins use Aesculus (horsamiut) Homeopathic.

Charcoal also helps in varicose veins.

Homeopathic Carduus Marianus (St. Mary's thistle) has also been known to help varicose veins.

Take cottage cheese and spread it on a cloth like you would spread butter on bread. Cover with another cloth and apply over aching and unsightly veins, if possible all night or just several hours. do this every night until gone.

For varicose veins or ulcers on the legs, apply hot sage compresses. Use sage tea on the leg and take frequent sage foot baths. Sage is also thought to improve a weak spine.

Varicose veins need zinc supplements.

— Vertigo —

Use crab apples for vertigo.

— Viral Infections —

Use romaine lettuce for viral infections.

Cinnamon is used for fighting viral and infectious diseases. Virus, bacteria, and fungus cannot live in the presence of cinnamon oil. It is helpful for chills, colds, and arthritis.

Lettuce water is an excellent remedy for a virus infection. Take leaf lettuce and boil in water. Drink four ounces every hour. Lettuce water can be applied externally over swollen parts of the body such as ankles, abdomen, and liver.

For viral infections in blood and lymph, use Homeopathic Echinacea.

It is known that nettle has anti-fungal and anti-viral properties.

Calendula tea can also be helpful in viral infections.

Chick-peas are also anti-viral, particularly for anti-polio virus.

An unbelievable healing process was found in olive tree leaves. In 1962, scientists reported that it was the chemical Oleuropein present in every leaf that made this plant so powerful. Later on, a chemical called Elonolican was found, and both these chemicals are powerful viral, viroid, retro-virus, and protozoan antidotes.

~ Vitamins ~

Alfalfa seeds are loaded with vitamin C. Alfalfa contains many trace minerals and, when used as a tea, releases pain in the head and limbs. If you sprout alfalfa seed and eat 2 tablespoons of sprouts twice a day, it will lower your cholesterol. Alfalfa stimulates the appetite and improves di-gestion. It is a very good mineral supplier and helps make the bowels move.

~ Vomiting ~

*see also Nausea, Travel Sickness

In cases of severe vomiting, moisten a cloth with warm vinegar and apply to the abdomen.

Cinnamon is good for vomiting.

Nutmeg also aids vomiting.

~ Warts ~

Use lemon peel for calluses, corns, or warts. Put the lemon peel (white side down) on afflicted area and cover with a Band-Aid to hold it in place overnight. Every night, put on a fresh piece of lemon peel.

Soak fenugreek seed in water until it makes a mucilage-like ointment. Apply to the wart and let dry. Use once a day until the wart disappears.

For warts on hands and face, use Homeopathic Dulcamara.

Treatment of warts should include topical application of cashew nut (Anacardium occidentale), oil of yellow cedar (Thuja occidentalis), and milk-weed juice. There are commercial wart removal kits available from your pharmacy that employ salicylic acid topically.

An old Native American cure recommends doctoring the wart three times a day with the milky substance found in the stems of dandelion and milkweed.

Apply a few drops of castor oil to wart and bandage tightly. Repeat procedure two or three times daily until wart disappears.

~ Water-Logged Tissues ~

*see also Bloated Condition, Fluid Retention

Banana is a good potassium fruit. Therefore, if taken in moderation, it will balance excess water in the system and is proved to be good for water-logged tissues. Bananas are also excellent for colitis, leucorrhea, backache, bulk producer, and diuretic.

Don't eat bananas if you have a cold, sniffles, coryza, or a cough. This will add to your problems. A banana baked in the skin, mashed with a little fresh cream or olive oil and made into a compress aids in swollen tonsils.

– Weakness –

Drink two cups of yarrow tea a day for weakness in senior citizens.

Arrowroot is a food for the weak, debilitated, and those who are convalescing. It is very easily digested, creating no gastric upset.

Dried apple peelings made into a tea are full of silicon and will strengthen muscles and improve other kinds of weaknesses.

– Wound Healing –

Nutrients that aid wound healing are:

zinc
vitamin C
vitamin E

Also arginine and amino acids enhance wound healing (*Americas Journal of Clinical Nutrition*).

Leg Ulcers:

Take two ounces of mulberry twigs and cut them into little pieces. Boil the pieces in one quart of grape juice for thirty minutes. Swish 1 table-spoon 6 times a day in your mouth before swallowing it. Two quarts should do.

Naturally Occurring Disease-Fighting Substances in Food

Also called phyto chemicals and functional foods.

Food	Active Ingredient
Apricots	Carotenoids
Basil	Monoterpenes
Beets	Anti-carcinogenic hormone
Berries	Catechins Flavonoids Phenolic acids
Broccoli	Monoterpenes Phenolic acid Plant sterols
Brussels sprouts	Indoles
Cabbage	Flavonoids Indoles Phenolic acids Plant sterols
Cantaloupe	Carotenoids
Carrots	Carotenoids Coumarins Flavonoids Monoterpenes Phenolic acids Phthalides Polyacetylenes

Celery	Phthalides
	Polyacetylenes
Citrus Fruits	Carotenoids
	Coumarins
	Flavonoids
	Monoterpenes
	Phenolic acid
	Triterpenoids
Cucumbers	Flavonoids
	Monoterpenes
	Plant sterols
Eggplant	Flavonoids
	Monoterpenes
	Phenolic acids
	Plant sterols
Flax seed	Alpha-linolenic acid
Grains (whole)	Phenolic acids
	Plant sterols
Grapefruit (red)	Lycopene
Green tea	Catechins
Horseradish	Isothiniocyanates
Kale	Carotenoids
	Indoles
Licorice root extract	Triterpenoids
Mint	Monoterpenes
Mustard	Isothiniocyanates

Parsley	Carotenoids
	Coumarins
	Flavonoids
	Monoterpenes
	Phenolic acids
	Phthalides
	Polyacetylenes
Peppers	Flavonoids
	Monoterpenes
	Phenolic acids
	Plant sterols
Radish	Isothiniocyanates
Soy products	Alpha-linolenic acid
	Flavonoids
	Plant sterols
	Triterpenoids
Spinach	Carotenoids
Squash	Flavonoids
	Monoterpenes
	Plant sterols
Sweet potatoes	Carotenoids
Tomatoes	Flavonoids
	Lycopene
	Monoterpenes
	Phenolic acid
	Plant sterols
Turnip greens	Carotenoids
Walnuts	Alpha-linolenic acid

Winter squash	Carotenoids
Yams	Carotenoids
	Flavonoids
	Monoterpenes
	Plant sterols

~ Food Combinations ~

Food Energies:

Eat for energy! Use your pendulum to determine positive, negative, and neutral foods and food combinations. Always beat/stir your food clockwise.

Apples:	It is neutral and goes with everything. Good to "eat an apple a day."
Apple Skin:	It has osmium, which is food for the brain. Make apple skin tea for kids before they go to school, and the kids will learn better. Affects the brain and nervous system.
Bread & Veggies:	Good combination.
Coffee:	It is neutral. When milk is added, it becomes negative. Same with white sugar. If honey is added, it becomes positive. If tired in the morning, take a cup of coffee with honey to open up all the glands. No more than 1 cup a day.
Eggshell:	Easily assimilated calcium. Put eggshells in apple cider vinegar and drink after they dissolve.

Fasts:	Never fast more than 3–4 days, because too many chemicals in the body will go deeper and deeper into the bone marrow. A good Native American fast: Day 1: Eat only fruit, except no bananas. Day 2: Drink only 1 gallon of hyssop tea to clean out lymph system. Day 3: Steamed vegetables only, cleans out intestines. Day 4: One gallon of mineral broth to clean out the lymph system.
Fruit & Veggies:	No energy.
Grains:	Too much can cause allergies.
Meat & Bread:	No energy when combined. It will take at least 2 hours for energy to return. Cheese and/or eggs with bread the same.
Meat & Potato:	Good combination.
Oats:	Keeps immune system going.
Peas:	Separate from other vegetables, especially carrots.
Rice:	Universal, neutral food. But it is not a protein.

Tomato:

Take out the core of the tomato, since the core is negative. The tomato is positive. Eat 2–3 times a week. For a tumor in the head, blend tomatoes and put on head as a poultice between 2 layers of cloth and the tumor will disappear.

Books by Hanna

"Wholistic health represents an attitude toward well being which recognizes that we are not just a collection of mechanical parts, but an integrated system which is physical, mental, social and spiritual."

Ageless Remedies from Mother's Kitchen

You will laugh and be amazed at all that you can do in your own pharmacy, the kitchen. These time tested treasures are in an easy to read, cross referenced guide. (92 pages)

Allergy Baking Recipes

Easy and tasty recipes for cookies, cakes, muffins, pancakes, breads and pie crusts. Includes wheat free recipes, egg and milk free recipes (and combinations thereof) and egg and milk substitutes. (34 pages)

Alzheimer's Science and God

This little booklet provides a closer look at this disease and presents Hanna's unique, religious perspectives on Alzheimer's disease. (15 pages)

Arteriosclerosis and Herbal Chelation

A booklet containing information on Arteriosclerosis causes, symptoms and herbal remedies. An introduction to the product *Circu Flow*. (14 pages)

Cancer: Traditional and New Concepts

A fascinating and extremely valuable collection of theories, tests, herbal formulas and special information pertaining to many facets of this dreaded disease. (65 pages)

Cookbook for Electro-Chemical Energies

The opening of this book describes basic principles of healthy eating along with some fascinating facts you may not have heard before. The rest of this book is loaded with delicious, healthy recipes. A great value. (106 pages)

God Helps Those Who Help Themselves

This work is a beautifully comprehensive description of the seven basic physical causes of disease. It is wholistic information as we need it now. A truly valuable volume. (196 pages)

Good Health Through Special Diets

This book shows detailed outlines of different diets for different needs. Dr. Reidlin, M.D. said, "The road to health goes through the kitchen not through the drug store," and that's what this book is all about. (90 pages)

Hanna's Workshop

A workbook that brings together all of the tools for applying Hanna's testing methods. Designed with 60 templates that enable immediate results.

How to Counteract Environmental Poisons

A wonderful collection of notes and information gleaned from many years of Hanna's teachings. This concise and valuable book discusses many toxic materials in our environment and shows you how to protect yourself from them. It also presents Hanna's insights on how to protect yourself, your family and your community from spiritual dangers. (53 pages)

Instant Herbal Locator

This is the herbal book for the do-it-yourself person. This book is an easy cross referenced guide listing complaints and the herbs that do the job. Very helpful to have on hand. (109 pages)

Instant Vitamin-Mineral Locator

A handy, comprehensive guide to the nutritive values of vitamins and minerals. Used to determine bodily deficiencies of these essential elements and combinations thereof, and what to do about these deficiencies. According to your symptoms, locate your vitamin and mineral needs. A very helpful guide. (55 pages)

New Dimensions in Healing Yourself

The consummate collection of Hanna's teachings. An unequated volume that compliments all of her other books as well as her years of teaching. (150 pages)

Old-Time Remedies for Modern Ailments

A collection of natural remedies from Eastern and Western cultures. There are 20 fast cleansing methods and many ways to rebuild your health. A health classic. (105 pages)

Parasites: The Enemy Within

A compilation of years of Hanna's studies with parasites. A rare treasure and one of the efforts to expose the truths that face us every day. (62 pages)

The Pendulum, the Bible and Your Survival

A guide booklet for learning to use a pendulum. Explains various aspects of energies, vibrations and forces. (22 pages)

The Seven Spiritual Causes of Ill Health

This book beautifully reveals how our spiritual and emotional states have a profound effect on our physical well being. It addresses fascinating topics such as karma, gratitude, trauma, laughter as medicine . . . and so much more. A wonderful volume full of timeless treasures. (142 pages)

Spices to the Rescue

This is a great resource for how our culinary spices can enrich our health and offer first aid from our kitchen. Filled with insightful historical references. (64 pages)

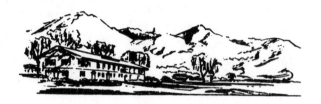

Peaceful Meadow Retreat

You are invited . . . .
to participate in the upcoming

NATURAL AND VIBRATIONAL HEALING SEMINARS

If you would like to learn how to help yourselves and others with exciting new healing methods, then these weekends are for you.

Learn unusual healing techniques from Hanna Kroeger, well-known lecturer and author of many books.

You will be taught the seven physical and spiritual causes of ill health and about such diseases as Candida albicans, Epstein-Barr and hidden nerve viruses which lower the immune system, MS, Alzheimer's disease and many others.

- Amazing discoveries in natural healing.
- The best learning vacation you ever had.

Rev. Rudolf and Hanna Kroeger
7075 Valmont Drive
Boulder, Colorado 80301
(303) 442-2490 or 443-0755